Bridging the Sex Addiction Divide

Mindful Considerations for Vulnerable Clients

by Dr. Michael Salas, PsyD, LPC-S, CSAT-S, CST

SANO PRESS

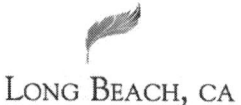

LONG BEACH, CA

Copyright © 2019 by Michael J. Salas
All rights reserved. This book or any portion thereof may not be reproduced or used in any manner whatsoever without the express written permission of the publisher except for the use of brief quotations in a book review.
Front image credit: "Sea Bridge" by Fradellafra (Pixabay) in accordance with Creative Commons CCO.

Printed in the United States of America
First Printing, 2018
ISBN-13: 978-1-7339222-3-4

Vantage Point Counseling Services
3300 Oak Lawn Ave, Ste 601
Dallas, TX 75219

vantagepointdallascounseling.com

I want to thank my husband, Michael, who is always supportive of my ambitions and goals.

I also want to thank my team at Vantage Point Counseling Services. I learn, inspire, am inspired by, and grow with you every day.

Contents

Introduction   1

Understanding the Sex Addiction Controversy   18

    How Extreme Division Impacts Our Field and Our Clients   19

    The Importance of Finding Balance Between Therapist Communities   29

    Beyond Labels and Moving Forward   56

    Working Towards Balance in Perspectives   60

Identifying the Problem   62

    Shame, Vulnerability, Connection and Addiction   76

    Five Points to Divide the Lines on Sex Addiction   81

    Vulnerable Groups   90

    Bridging the Divide: Putting Down Weapons and Armor to Help Those in Need   93

Considerations for Sexual Orientation and Gender   96

    Sex Addiction Therapy with LGBTQ Clients   100

    Concerns for Gay and Lesbian Clients and Sexual Compulsivity   118

    Considerations for Bisexual Clients   122

    Navigating Heteronormativity and Cisgender Bias   123

    Mixed-Orientation Marriages   126

    Overcoming Your Biases   128

    Special Considerations for Transgender and Gender Non-Binary Individuals   137

Considerations for Kink, BDSM, and "Fetishes"   154

The Shame in Labels and What to Consider	155
Relationships, Boundaries, and Self-Expression	158
The Dynamics of Holding Space for Kink, BDSM, and Fetishes	163
Infidelity in Kink, BDSM, and "Fetishes"	167
How Trauma Therapy Can Help Rather than Hinder	170
Building a Foundation with Trust	171
The Lines of Compulsivity	173
Sex Positive Considerations for Kink, "Fetishes," and BDSM	177

Considerations for Non-Monogamy — 185

Boundaries, Relationships, and Communication	188
The Importance of Grounding and Foundational Support	197
Infidelity and Sexual Compulsivity in Non-Monogamy	199
Drawing the Lines of Addiction in Non-Monogamy	202
Sex Positive Therapy for Non-Monogamy	211
Sex Addiction and Non-Monogamy	214

Mindful Sex Addiction Therapy and Beyond — 217

Sex Positive Rules	218
Asking versus Telling	237
Accepting Client Struggles as Growth	244
Mindfulness and Centering	246

Conclusion — 260

References and Resources — 264

Introduction

Every year, thousands of people seek out help for problems with compulsive sexual behavior. Some of them have a genuine problem with behavior that has become out of control. Others aren't addicts, but instead are responding to sexual shame and cultural issues. There is a lot of middle ground on this issue.

In the psychotherapy community, this topic is often confusing, contentious, and controversial. Sex addiction is often painted as if it has to be an "either/or" issue: you either believe in it or not. Like most controversies, it's far too complex to view it from such oversimplified and extreme perspectives.

The term "sex addiction" resonates with some people, while it angers and confuses others. This label often leads to intense debates among therapists and confusion among potential clients. These discussions, along with a lack of consensus on the topic, have a huge impact on many of our clients. In this book, I'll explore these controversies and discuss considerations to help our clients in a balanced way.

Before I begin, I want to take some time to share a little bit about my own experiences with these controversies. As a Certified Sex

Addiction Therapist (CSAT) and Certified Sex Therapist (CST), I've seen these arguments up close, from various points-of-view. But I didn't begin my career as either a CSAT or a CST, and so my experiences with sex addiction didn't start with the training from either of these certifications. Like most therapists, I started out as someone who simply wanted to help others. I'm guessing this is also true for the majority of the therapists who are reading this book. I hold onto the passion for helping clients who are brave enough to enter my therapy office. My hope is that this book will help them by being a resource for you, the therapist.

First of all, let me explain why I believe it's important to share a little bit about my professional story. I think it will resonate with many who read this book. I hope this book can help therapists identify when the sex addiction label is important and necessary, and when it isn't. Additionally, I hope that this book can assist therapists in helping clients who are vulnerable to shame and stigma.

Another big hope is that this book can help you view sex addiction through a balanced lens. This can be difficult to do. I hope that sharing a little piece of my story can help you understand why I believe that balance is important. Although I imperfectly manage this balance every day, I really believe that working towards this is critical to helping our clients. This is especially true of clients who are dealing with sexual compulsivity.

Balance is also professionally important. It helps us listen and learn from others with whom we don't really agree. It also helps us question ourselves, which I believe is critical when helping those who are vulnerable. I will be getting into managing this balance later in this book. But first, let me tell you how I came to the conclusion that this book was needed.

When I began my career in therapy, my primary specialty was in substance abuse. It didn't take long for me to realize that substance abuse therapy involved more than working with problems relating to alcohol and drugs. Anxiety, depression, anger, attachment issues, and trauma were very common things that surrounded and fed into these issues. I felt well-equipped to help my clients with the majority of their problems—even this early on in my career.

Despite my successes, I felt as if I was lacking in one arena. Sexuality was a common issue that came up during my sessions with several of my clients, and I didn't quite know how to help. As a gay man, this was troubling to me. One of my dreams was always to turn therapy into a space where clients could holistically process through their challenges. Yet, there was an integral part of their lives that I felt ill-equipped to help with. Looking back now, I'm sure that sexuality issues were even more common than I identified at that time. A lot of people don't bring these issues up when they're talking with their therapists. I obviously never intentionally ignored sexuality in therapy, but I'm sure that my inexperience allowed some information to go unnoticed.

When it came to sexuality, one issue repeatedly came up in therapy. Several of my clients reported struggling with compulsive sexual behavior. For them, the behavior was out of control, it was interfering with their lives, and they had no idea what to do about it. Some were isolating themselves with porn. Others were cheating. Some were putting their careers at risk.

Despite how much I wanted to help, I felt limited in my ability. I often felt frustrated in these clients' outcomes. Those who were dealing with sexual compulsivity just weren't improving as consistently as my other clients. I felt stuck.

Despite my frustration, I did notice trends in these clients. Many were struggling in their relationships. Some of them had serious problems connecting to their partners and would compulsively watch porn. Others would sexually chat with people and reported wasting hours isolating themselves from their families. Finally, there were clients who compulsively cheated. They knew that they were hurting themselves and their families, but couldn't stop.

I could tell that many of these clients were mired in a loop and they authentically wanted to find a way out. They didn't know where to begin their journey of change. I didn't really know where to start with it either. I really only had minimal success with the skills that were working with other clients who had other issues.

In retrospect, I needed training that would help me conceptualize these cases. With a better understanding of the dynamics behind the behavior, I would've been better able to intervene. Back then, I was also only trained in short-term therapy approaches. Although these interventions did help clients manage some of their symptoms, they would often return to therapy a few months to a year after treatment had ended. This was different from those cases that we all have, where clients return to therapy to work on new goals. Instead, they came back with the same issues. Sometimes their issues were even more severe.

I eventually moved to Dallas and started my own private practice. It wasn't long before I started receiving calls from men who were struggling with sexually compulsive behavior. However, many of these potential clients would contact me with a specific request. They would specifically ask if I was a Certified Sex Addiction Therapist (CSAT). In fact, several of them told me that they had previously tried working with a therapist who didn't have this credential, and it wasn't a good experience.

I've been a therapist in a variety of settings over the years. I know that there are a lot of non-CSAT therapists who do wonderful work with clients who are living with sex addiction and problematic sexual behaviors. I also know that credentials don't necessarily make therapists good at what they do; however, when clients consistently send a message, it's important to listen. Or at least, it's important to get more information. When it came to this credential, the message was clear: people felt they needed evidence of their therapist's ability to treat sexually compulsive behavior.

As with any training, practitioners have to find a way to make it their own. My experience was that the CSAT training provided very useful information regarding the conceptualization of sex addiction cases. The training offered tools for identifying sex addiction, as well as tools to help clients on their way through their recovery journey. This certification process also included coursework that analyzed client cases with more depth, which was something that I needed at that point in my career.

After obtaining the CSAT credential, sexual addiction became a primary focus of my work. I worked with individuals and couples on rebuilding trust, managing out-of-control behaviors, and identifying the sources of their problems. I saw significant improvement in my clients' abilities to work through these issues. They learned how to manage their behaviors and how to co-exist with their partners. However, I also noticed that there was yet another barrier for these clients. Several of them struggled to step back into sexual intimacy. In fact, some of them even admitted that they had never felt comfortable with sex in their relationships.

I was comfortable with helping these clients open up a dialogue to reestablish sexual relationships, but again, they often got stuck in another plateau. I worked on getting more training in trauma therapies, thinking that this would equip me with skills to help my clients with sexual intimacy. This training did help. Even still, I felt like something was still missing from my repertoire.

To better help these clients, I dove head first into another certification process to become a sex therapist. I believed that this education would help me assist couples in rekindling their sexual connections. I also knew that this certification could compliment skills from other trainings to help with trauma, infidelity, and betrayal.

What I didn't expect when becoming a CST was the depth of the controversy surrounding sex addiction. Before I get into this, let me take a step back. Being a gay male, it has always been important to me to provide a space that would help clients accept themselves. I also have to point out that I'm not bias-free or without flaws. I continue to grow and learn every day. We'll be talking about personal biases and values systems a lot in this book. I believe the most important antidote to bias is personal awareness.

On my journey to earning the CST credential, I had a blind spot about sex addiction therapy. I had some awareness of the historical issues surrounding sex addiction, especially as they related to the

Lesbian, Gay, Bisexual, Transgender, and Queer (LGBTQ) community. However, I never anticipated how negative the feelings were about sex addiction among critics of the label. I was also surprised by how intense the emotions were surrounding the CSAT credential itself.

Over the years, I watched the emotions surrounding sex addiction and the CSAT credential intensify. In particular, I saw the divide between CSTs and CSATs become more prominent. I also witnessed both communities further label, judge, and criticize each other. My stress levels increased as I wondered if I would have to choose between these credentials and communities.

CSATs were often labeled as close-minded, religious, and prudish zealots. On the other hand, CSTs were often stereotyped as professionals who promoted unhealthy sexual boundaries. As time passed, there was less and less common ground between these groups. Sadly, discussions about sex addiction were becoming lower, nastier, and more immature. At one especially heated point in this professional divide, I was shocked when people of color and the LGBTQ community were being used to promote talking points for one side of the debate on sex addiction. I need to point out that this conversation lacked open representation of people of color and LGBTQ individuals. When I tried to interject with perspectives as a gay, Latinx male, there was little interest in discussing the depth of the issue any further. In other words, the conversation wasn't about representing these groups at all; rather these groups were only being used as tools to argue and debate.

Several discussions on sex addiction have led to the questioning of politics, morality, talent, and intelligence of therapists who are on the other side of the debate. This energy has permeated well beyond these discussions as well. Whether it has been on social media, in written articles, or in general comments, I've heard therapists on both sides make incorrect, hurtful, and judgmental statements about therapists who have different perspectives on sex addiction.

At that point I remember thinking, "This is all such bullshit." I know brilliant and talented people on both sides of this argument. I couldn't understand why disagreements had to become so extreme. Even worse, I saw this impacting my clients. Several of them focused more and more on what so-called experts believed about the label, rather than focusing on their perspectives of their own problems.

I have several concerns about how low the conversations about sex addiction have sunk amongst therapists. I'm even more concerned about how the therapy communities' handling of this topic has impacted our clients. I believe that unbalanced professional opinions on this topic oversimplify our clients and their lives.

I embarked on my own journey to find a balance. I've worked to hear people on both sides, without giving up my own perspectives in the process. Sometimes I've succeeded, while other times I've failed. Either way, I believe that I've identified some of the most significant ways of growing as a profession and keeping our clients as the focus of psychotherapy, without falling victim to bullshit assumptions about sex addiction and the professionals who work with this problem.

As read this book, you will notice a balancing act. I will encourage you to hold a mirror up to your clients, and allow them to interpret what they see. I will push you to do this more than sitting in the expert position in your sessions. There are times when we need to be experts, but most times clients will identify with what resonates with them, regardless of our therapeutic opinions. For us to help with this process, we have to find a middle ground. This can be extremely challenging, but I believe that not doing this negatively impacts the people we work with. As you'll read later in this book, I believe that it impacts people who are the most vulnerable.

Finding Balance by Searching for the Middle Ground

Being a part of communities with polarized opinions on sex addiction has been challenging. I'm sure it will be challenging for several of you who are reading this as well. It's been hard work to identify my middle ground and personal understanding of my relationship with therapy for sex addiction. This book has been part of that process for me.

Over the years, I've learned a lot from members of both the American Association of Sexuality Educators, Counselors, and Therapists (AASECT) and International Institute for Trauma and Addiction Professionals (IITAP) communities. I've witnessed several discussions up close on my journey with both communities. I've learned about the passion that is behind these conversations and I know how meaningful these conversations are. I also know that there are several different backgrounds, personal experiences, and even professions that represent both sides of this debate. All of these experiences and perspectives matter, yet they can get drowned out by the intense fighting. This is what inspired me to write this book. I wanted to find a middle ground.

Bridging the Divide in a Polarized Time

Since I started writing this book, our political and cultural climate has become increasingly intense. What divides us has become even more magnified. I believe that these divisions have increased the polarization between proponents and critics of sex addiction. This is because social and cultural concerns are at the heart of many of the debates surrounding sex addiction.

When it comes to sex addiction therapy, I have witnessed professional discussions transform from listening and sharing into pontification, name-calling, labeling, threats, slander, and unfair criticisms. I have even seen disagreements deteriorate into Internet trolling and threats of litigation.

No one wants to be on the receiving end of any of this behavior. There is a dynamic to this controversy that is similar to the polarized breakdown that we see in our country right now. Similar to how you're expected to pick political sides, you're expected to pick sides on the sex addiction debate. From this perspective, it doesn't matter whether you use facts to back up your arguments either. Instead, it's much more important that you "fit in" with one side or the other.

Here are the polarized undertones I've noticed from both sides of the sex addiction debate:

- You better jump to conclusions about those who disagree with you.
- Facts don't necessarily matter.
- You can only belong on one side of this debate.
- Domination and power are more important than compromise.

- No one should have to tolerate opinions that differ from their own.
- If you disagree with someone, you get to say anything you want about them, without verifying whether it's true or not.

Yes, it's true—This type of behavior is displayed by therapists. It's displayed by the same professionals who are supposed to help clients rediscover balance, reconnection, and work through the crises in their lives.

I also understand that therapists are human beings. Our humanity will be another major focus of this book. We screw up. The problem is less about the "screw ups" and more about stubbornness and failure to take responsibility.

This behavior also pushes a large portion of professional voices to the fringes. Don't believe me? I've been backchanneled enough to know that therapists don't feel safe to disagree with the norms of their peers. This is true of the AASECT and sex addiction communities. I've been told by therapists that when they disagree, they risk being called dumb, bigoted, ignorant, and even personally unaware. They can be called sex-negative as well. I've heard therapists get called close-minded and uncaring. Criticism has even gone as far as labeling professionals who disagree as "bad."

I believe it's critical that therapists learn how to tolerate dialogue on this topic. Without these conversations, there are several consequences. One of the biggest consequences is that closed-mindedness oversimplifies sociocultural issues.

When opinions are shared on sexual health, politics are likely to become part of the discussion. Sex and politics are almost always intertwined. Therapist communities are struggling to identify how to have these conversations. As a result, many of these discussions are avoided altogether. Even worse, these conversations can quickly turn into public shaming, ridicule, and even slander.

I'm in this field because I love to help my clients. I don't believe that professionals who refuse to listen to other professionals or regulate themselves on controversial topics can effectively help their clients. In fact, a lot of the work that we do with our clients is to help them tolerate differences while continuing to openly communicate.

When therapists behave in this way, psychotherapy becomes wrongfully focused on the therapists. The focus turns more and more towards filling the egos of so-called "experts." This is unnecessarily confusing to our clients. We need to stay grounded to our roles. Our clients are complex and by oversimplifying this debate to the existence and non-existence of sex addiction, we're not respecting all of the dynamics that our clients bring to our offices.

Both critics and proponents of sex addiction can help clients who are dealing with sexually compulsive behavior. Success has more to do with clients' perspectives of their problems and trust in their therapists, than it has to do with their therapists' opinions on this problem. I'm aware of how important therapeutic skills are because they can largely influence relationships and trust. However, there is no sexuality organization that holds a trademark on these interpersonal skills.

I'm not saying that there is no place to scientifically study the impact of the sex addiction label. There is certainly a place for science. For the purpose of this book, I will be focusing the complexities and delicate issues that occur in sex addiction cases. To be more specific, I'll be focusing on the dynamics that likely play a role in your therapy sessions. Several of my peers and friends in the field have asked me important questions about sexually compulsive behavior over the years. Most of these questions have revolved around vulnerable groups and populations who are at risk of being shamed. These therapists are interested in building the relationships that are needed for therapeutic success.

"Is My Client Dealing with a Sex Addiction or Not?"

Therapists who strive to be sex positive can struggle with identifying the separation between sex addiction and non-addictive sexual, relationship, and gender expression. It's a struggle because the lines become blurry. For clinical enthusiasts who are reading this book, it's tempting to search for simplified definitions of sex addiction. I get it. It would make everything easier to understand, including sex addiction. However, simplification isn't the purpose of this book. In fact, oversimplification of this issue has contributed to division. There are too many sociocultural issues surrounding sex and gender to make sex addiction so oversimplified.

I believe that diagnostic labels are limited in their benefits to our clients. They can help us conceptualize cases, but they usually become less important as we get to know our clients. The process is what eventually takes center stage. Some clients find comfort in diagnostic labels. In these situations, diagnoses help them understand their problems, share their stories, and find supportive communities.

In writing this book, I tried to identify rules that could always be used to identify a sex addiction. I knew that this would make working with the groups discussed in this book easier. Unfortunately,

I never identified rules that can be applied in every case. I believe this is true of all clinical problems.

Rather than focusing on specific rules, I've identified considerations for mindfulness. When working with the groups discussed in this book, it's almost impossible to deal with sexual problems without also addressing historical issues with religion, morality, health, and/or social norms. These things are complex. When it comes to vulnerable groups and sex addiction, these complex issues must be considered in order to be sex positive. At the same time, I don't believe that specific rules can be written, because people are too complex for this. The way that our clients identify with these potential concerns is very individualistic. We have to respect their personal reflections and expressed therapeutic needs.

Vulnerable Groups in Sex Addiction Therapy

There are specific groups that are commonly discussed in the sex addiction controversy. The primary concern in the controversy is that the sex addiction label shames members of these groups. Without caution, this concern can become a reality. These groups are vulnerable because they're at a higher risk of being shamed and judged. These negative interactions relate to our clients' relationship boundaries, sexual expression, gender, non-traditional desires, and sexual orientation.

We live in a culture that normalizes cis-genderism and heterosexuality. Therefore, LGBTQ clients are vulnerable in all therapy, but particularly when it comes to sex addiction therapy. These groups of people have a long history of being shamed and persecuted for who they are. This mistreatment continues today.

Conversion therapy, reparative therapy, and Sexual Orientation Change Efforts (SOCE) are more commonly viewed as unethical in our culture and in psychotherapy. Therapists who use SOCE also regularly claim that they're treating "sexual addictions." Although these practices are illegal in many states, they're still legal in most. This makes LGBTQ clients vulnerable to harm from such approaches.

Kink and Bondage & Discipline, Domination & Submission, and Sadomasochism (BDSM) have a long history of being classified as behavior problems and addictions. In my work with people from these groups, I believe there is an increased risk of shame as well. Relationships and sexual expressions classified as kink have often been labeled as sexual addictions. Out of shame, many of these clients seek out help for compulsive behavior when there is no compulsivity at all. When treated as an addiction, shame can increase, which promotes secrecy, poor boundaries, and mindlessness.

Similar to those who are involved in kink and BDSM, those who swing, are in open relationships, and who are polyamorous are also vulnerable during sex addiction treatment. Although our society has become more open-minded about non-monogamy, we live in a culture that still primarily promotes monogamous relationships. I've found that non-monogamy is often treated in therapy like it's something that's unhealthy. This can lead to serious issues that prevent clients from being open and developing their boundary systems.

These aren't the only groups who are vulnerable when it comes to sex addiction. However, advocacy for these groups has led to some of the most intense controversies. As someone who works hard to be a sex-positive therapist every day and who is a member of one of these groups, I wanted to write a book that would help therapists consider important factors in sex addiction when working with these groups.

Working with sex addiction and clients from these vulnerable groups can feel like a tight rope balancing act. Balancing on this rope can make this work difficult and even overwhelming. In the sex addiction divide, it can be risky to ask questions. This is why I encourage you to ask more questions of yourself throughout this book. I also encourage you to find supportive colleagues who will respect you while you ask them questions as well. I truly believe this approach can help you grow and provide the best support to your clients. But it won't be easy. I hope this book gives you some useful, basic information to consider along with tools that you can continue to use.

Who Should Read This Book?

This book is for open minds. Hopefully, it will help you walk into new, uncomfortable conversations with other therapists. If your agenda is domination of the therapy world, or to prove the existence or non-existence of sex addiction, I don't think you'll find much benefit from reading this. In this book, I encourage the disarming of therapists, not arming up.

This book is for therapists who are looking for sex-positive considerations in their work with sex addiction. While you're reading this, I will push you to look at yourself through a few different lenses. This will help you tackle your own biases, which I've found to be invaluable when helping my clients.

Finally, this book can help you learn about how groups can be vulnerable to mislabeling and what you can do about this vulnerability. Each chapter will discuss common biases and help you find ways to work through them. Yes, unfortunately, this will be an ongoing process. However, I hope that reading this will help you build a foundation for future work with your clients.

I appreciate you taking the time to read this book.

1

Understanding the Sex Addiction Controversy

Throughout this book, I'll be talking a lot about mindfulness and personal awareness. To practice this level of awareness, it's essential to understand the complexities of the sex addiction controversy. Without this understanding, it's easy to fall into the divide, which can increase your odds of negatively impacting your clients.

Along with the discussion on the controversies surrounding sex addiction, I'll also be discussing some of the history that has led to these controversies. In case you're not as familiar with sex addiction, this will give you some context of the origins of the debates, but also the intense emotions behind them. For the purposes of this book, I'll be focusing on more current hot topics on this issue; however, all of the controversies and issues in this book have long histories that I encourage you to read more about after you've finished this book. One great resource that really delves deep into the long backstory of sex addiction is *Sex Addiction as Affect Dysregulation* by Alexandra Katehakis.

Having a good understanding of all of the professional riffs regarding sex addiction can help you play many vital roles. First, it will help you professionally by finding a balance in professional discussions, without isolating yourself on the topic. It can help you avoid harmful assumptions about your peers. Most importantly, you'll be able to help your clients without causing them harm.

How Extreme Division Impacts Our Field and Our Clients

When it comes to sex addiction, the psychotherapy community is very much divided. Sexuality professionals, in particular, struggle to find a middle ground on this topic. Most therapists will encounter at least one client who comes into their office claiming to have a problem with compulsive, sexual behavior. Some of these people will have had multiple affairs. Others will disclose issues about compulsive pornography use. When so many seek out help for this problem, why is sex addiction still so controversial?

Past mistakes of the psychotherapy and sexuality fields have taken their toll. All psychotherapy subdivisions have professionals who fight to be known as leading experts. The fight for domination includes individual therapists, but it also involves entire organizations. If it sounds like this controversy is messy, it's because it involves so many people and organizations.

In this book, I'll explore several of the perspectives surrounding sex addiction. Some of these perspectives have transformed into extreme battles about the definitions of healthy sexuality. When you read these perspectives, you'll see how these opinions can turn into broad, unfair theories about sex and relationships. Even worse, you'll see how they can end up confusing and shaming our clients for their boundaries, needs, and desires.

Professional battles over the definitions of healthy sexuality create an illusion in our field. The illusion is that romantic and sexual relationships have strict, easy-to-follow definitions and rules that everyone should live by. This creates a cycle of ongoing problems in our field. Our field then sets a tone that we can define healthy sexuality for clients. Both clients and therapists fall for this myth. Therapists start defining these things for their clients. Overreaching definitions lead to shame. Our clients expect us to define healthy sexuality for them.

As you're probably already aware, these illusions play an enormous role on professional riffs surrounding sex addiction. Clients who are seeking out help for sex addiction are usually wanting to discover healthy sexuality in their lives. This makes them vulnerable to the harm of overreaching definitions of healthy sexuality. Here are some of the most common, harmful, and overreaching definitions that I have seen professionals use in sex addiction cases:

- Pornography is always bad.
- All men watch porn and women need to deal with it.
- Toys and sexual aids are unhealthy.
- Masturbation is unhealthy.
- Kink is dangerous and unhealthy.
- Cheating is inevitable, and all people should just open their relationships.
- Sex outside of marriage is always immoral.
- Sexually fluid people are really just confused.
- People are usually too uptight about sex.

As we get deeper into this book, you'll see that this list is far from complete. In each section, I'll do my best to name different perspectives and definitions along with their potential outcomes.

For now, I want to discuss how extreme opinions on sexuality are harmful. When we oversimplify complex disagreements, it can lead to dichotomies. These extremes create sides on topics that should be open to discussion. In fact, opinions on sex addiction are now primarily on two opposite, rigid ends of a contentious spectrum.

When professionals share their opinions on sex addiction, they're assigned to a group. They're perceived as antagonists or protagonists. There are four dichotomies that are commonly used to categorize therapists who are on either side of this controversy. In these dichotomies, you'll see fertile ground for judgment and assumptions. You won't see much room for openness either. Instead, people are assigned to a category that questions their intelligence, self-awareness, and even morality. This prevents open discussions about sex addiction. Here are the four primary, dichotomous ways that therapists categorize each other when discussing this topic:

1. Good vs. Bad
2. Healthy vs. Unhealthy
3. Worthy vs. Unworthy
4. Smart vs. Dumb

These extremes ignore the complexities of human sexuality, as well as the individual stories of our clients. They're disrespectful to colleagues. They also prevent discussions that can lead to better theories of treatment for sexual compulsivity.

These dichotomies create another professional illusion. This is the illusion that therapists are all-knowing sexuality experts. I don't call this an illusion because therapists have no knowledge. Your opinions on sexuality matter. We have all read, studied, and taken courses to build our opinions. I call this an illusion because the importance of the expertise of therapists is inflated by our culture and even our field. Therapy is all about the client process. The war to be experts is about therapist egos, domination, and monopolization. When therapists use dichotomous labeling, they're viewing therapists who have different opinions as opponents. Sometimes they're even viewing them as enemies. In these situations, therapists are oversimplifying sexuality, gender, and relationships.

There are several ways to help our clients. Of course, there are some lines that can always be drawn. I'll be naming a few of these boundaries throughout this book. For the moment, I want to draw a larger focus onto the importance of the nuances of helping our clients. When we fall into dichotomous labeling, we're at risk of bulldozing our clients' perceptions about their own stories. All-knowing experts don't have to listen because they already know the algorithms of all human behavior. This way of thinking is toxic and it doesn't help our clients.

When clients come into our offices for help with sexual compulsivity, they're dealing with a variety of issues. You'll start conceptualizing your case from the moment you take the inquiry on the phone. It's almost impossible for therapists to avoid this. In fact, this conceptualization is important when screening our clients to determine whether or not we can help them. Your conceptualization is going to reflect your opinions. I don't expect you to erase them.

Instead, I want you to be aware of them so that you can remain cautious of how you process your theories with your clients.

It takes a lot of courage for our clients to contact us. Many of us have made those calls to therapists ourselves. We're aware of how difficult it is to pick a professional to talk to. This is a vulnerable time for our clients. If we make one wrong move at this point in the process, we can push the client away. Therefore, we have to know when to share our conceptualizations with them.

Expert opinions work well in books, articles, blogs, and on television. However, clients don't need clinicians to define healthy sexuality for them. Most of them have had too much of others defining this for them already in their lives. Instead, they need someone who will help them identify their problems for themselves and help them find ways of navigating through their life journeys.

All of this being said, the controversy about sex addiction isn't without merit. Clients are often prematurely labeled as sex addicts by therapists. When clients are concerned about possible compulsive sexual behaviors, there are several other issues that can lead to incorrect labeling as well. Some clients are responding to religious shame when they come into therapy for sex addiction. Others are mislabeled as sex addicts when they are struggling with self-acceptance of their authentic desires, orientation, or gender. Sadly, this over-labeling continues to happen to this day.

Balance is needed when working with clients who seek out therapy for sex addiction, whether the label is appropriate or not. These situations can be complicated, and I've found that therapists are often at risk of oversimplifying cases to fit their opinions on sexuality and gender. There are several therapists who strip the label of addiction from their clients. I've seen the opposite take place as well. There are just as many therapists who have labeled client behaviors as addictive even when the label was inappropriate.

When client perspectives are harshly invalidated, they may prematurely leave therapy. We're working in an era with more sophisticated clients. They have often already researched their problems way before they come to our offices. Of course, there are limitations in self-diagnosing, but when a problem or label resonates with a client, therapists need to listen. Rather than using self-diagnosis as an opportunity to invalidate, therapists can use the process of self-diagnosis as clinical information. We don't have to agree with our clients. However, our job is to help them identify interpersonal and psychosexual dynamics that are leading to problems in their lives.

When our clients are dealing with a crisis, they're going to be looking for constructs, labels, and prescriptions to make sense of the situation that they're in. A label such as sex addiction can make things easier for them to understand in a time of crisis. Partners of clients are sometimes the ones who believe that the sex addiction label fits their partner. Sometimes this label is appropriate, while other times it will miss the mark. Whether the label fits or not, the case is always much more complex than the debate over the existence of sex addiction.

There are many moving parts when people are dealing with issues that involve sex and relationships. All of this requires therapists to manage a careful balancing act. There are several people involved in these therapeutic processes, and all of them (clients and therapists) will have their perspectives on sexuality. That includes you too!

Now, let's start building (and rebuilding) a mindful foundation by getting into the underbelly of the sex addiction controversies.

Scratching the Surface of the Divide

The sex addiction controversy is quite complex and it runs deep. It includes several organizations, professionals, and various fields. The controversy has led to hurt feelings and misunderstandings. Fueling it are valid concerns about social and sexual constructs. For professionals who follow these debates, it might seem like you have to pick sides.

What is the origin of this division? It certainly didn't happen overnight. I believe the best way to help our clients is to mend the division. I don't mean that we all have to agree. Instead, I think the best way to help our clients is to find ways of respectfully disagreeing. In order to mend the division, it's important to understand the background of what got us here.

Labels, Perceptions, and Criticisms

Professionals in the field often believe that sexually compulsive behavior exists. However, they struggle with controversies about what to call these behavior patterns. The most commonly used labels are *sexual addiction, sexual compulsivity*, and *out-of-control sexual behavior*.

Then there are those who believe that the best label is no label at all. Professionals in this camp believe that sexual addiction doesn't exist. The arguments against the possible existence of sexually compulsive behavior vary. Some argue that science doesn't support the label. Other professionals insist that the behavior patterns are misinterpretations of other issues.

Some clients identify with the label, but there is a lot of criticism about this self-identification. Some critics believe that these people are repressing their sexual desires in a sexually rigid society. It's true, sexual shame and self-repression are evident in several clients who label their behaviors as addictive. When these people are offered sexual education and increased openness, they often discover an increased sense of personal, sexual authenticity. In these situations, some of these clients will find that the label of sex addiction never applied to them to begin with. While other clients continue to identify with it throughout their lives.

Finally, there are therapists who hold on tightly to the idea of "healthy" sexual behavior that matches their belief system. They have strong beliefs that clients need to abide by these rules of morality. Therapists in this group tend to believe that part of their position as professionals is to educate others about sexual health. However, this group doesn't solely base their ideas of sexual health on sexual consent and self-determination. Rather, they view their role as a gatekeeper of morality.

Sex Positivity and the Tension Surrounding Sex Addiction

I believe that one major source of tension between proponents and critics of sex addiction revolves around therapists' perceptions of superiority and morality. Some therapists promote sexual oppression and repression. Others shame their clients for not being as "free" and "sexually open" as they believe that their clients should be. All of these situations revolve around therapists projecting their belief systems onto their clients.

Sexual addiction has become associated (in this debate) with sexual oppression and repression. Some therapists have perpetuated this with their rigid and even oppressive definitions of healthy sexuality. What makes this worse is that these same therapists often insist that their clients must abide by these particular boundaries.

However, I've also seen therapists who push their clients in a different direction. These therapists have their own definitions of sex positivity and push their clients to be congruent with these beliefs and boundaries.

Belief systems are strong and powerful forces, even among therapists. This energy doesn't always lead to openness and generosity. It usually leads to the opposite. It opens up a pathway for rigidity and closed-mindedness. Rather than learning more about the perspectives of people who have different beliefs, professionals are actually being taught to grip to divisive truths. They're being taught that there is no middle ground. Yet, our clients often bring "middle-ground" situations, emotions, and relationship circumstances into our offices. These extremes are doing them a disservice.

Sexual Compulsivity vs. Out-of-Control Sexual Behavior vs. Sex Addiction

For many of our colleagues, the most controversial issue surrounding sex addiction is the term *sex addiction* itself. This isn't going to be a surprise to readers who are already members of either the sex addiction and/or sex therapy communities. There are professionals who believe that this term promotes a label that doesn't fit what clients are actually experiencing. They believe that suggesting such a label can be shaming. From this perspective, this shame can lead to more issues with sexuality, rather than fewer. And yes, I've seen this happen to clients, and we'll be talking about this throughout this book.

A lack of clarity is another problem that I believe is behind the debate on the sex addiction label. *Addiction* is generally a vague label. Mixed with concerns of shaming clients, many therapists have worked to identify terms they feel are more appropriate. Some therapists call these behaviors "sexually compulsive." Others call them "out-of-control sexual behaviors."

It's true that there are clients who benefit from stepping away from the use of the addiction label. They might be taking this label on to satisfy a loved one. Sometimes they use this because they feel incongruent with the religious perspectives of their sexual behavior. Others might use this label out of confusion about their sexuality. They might also be unsure of what they need, what they want, and the kind of help they're seeking.

Then there are those clients who are insistent that their patterns of behavior are an addiction. They might find some solace in Twelve Step communities. They find social support in these places when working through a relationship that is falling apart, and when they're dealing with the chaos that can come from deep, emotional pain. This support helps them get through their issues by supporting balance where things were once out of control.

Different perspectives from both professionals and clients make it difficult to find a balance in therapy. I believe this challenge has intensified the debate on sex addiction. We're in a field that teaches us that labels will lead us to the best possible treatment plans to help our clients. However, most of us have come to realize that labels don't do much holistically to help the people who are sitting in front of us in therapy.

Does this mean we should just get rid of the sex addiction label altogether? No, because the stories and experiences of our clients are most important. There are clients who identify their symptomology as an addiction. We'll be discussing more about addiction later in this book. First, we have to dive deeper into the spiraling controversy of sex addiction. Unfortunately, I'm just getting started in explaining how deep this controversy runs.

The Importance of Finding Balance Between Therapist Communities

The sexuality field is full of intelligent, articulate, and passionate people. In the case of sexual addiction, advocacy is mixed with passion. I love passion because it's what promotes change; however, when passion goes unchecked, it can destroy the much-needed dialogue that is required for growth. When it comes to the topic of sex addiction, this unregulated passion has created an atmosphere that is often void of professional respect because it's difficult to stay with facts when we feel this way.

Controversies over sex addiction aren't among the only riffs we've seen in psychotherapy subdivisions. Theoretical evolution always involves some amount of chaos. There is a common historical pattern of this in our field. Professionals stick to their ideology, dig their heels into their positions, and fight to prove that they were right all along. In time, these theoretical disagreements typically merge into new and better theories of the problem; though, it tends to take a lot of time and effort to reach this consensus. It also requires professionals to walk into territories of discomfort with open-mindedness.

These riffs don't only happen in psychology. For example, there's a similar polarization on the topic of diet and exercise in the medical field. Medical camps tend to hold strong opinions regarding the roles of sugar, dietary fat, and exercise in disease. Some believe that dietary fat makes you overweight and being overweight can lead to a long list of health problems. While others think that dietary fat shouldn't have been implicated in the first place. Instead, they believe it's actually sugar and carbohydrates that are the true causes of these health issues. Despite these strongly held positions by well-respected, intelligent, and reputable medical researchers and professionals, we still don't have a consensus. Instead, both sides work to prove that their perspectives are fact. Despite all of these arguments, here most of us are, still unclear on what the healthiest dietary plan should be.

Despite this long history, there is some evidence that medicine could be changing. Some research-based groups have pulled together different perspectives on this serious medical issue. By doing so, they can ask tough questions about past and current research. They can test out new theories. Finally, they can keep each other in check so that they can avoid extremes.

The field of sexuality deals with similar divisive dynamics on theories of sexual behavior. At this time, we're still very far from any consensus about sex addiction. There is little evidence that open minds or open ears will take center stage in this debate any time soon. The debate is primarily dominated by two sides, rather than reflecting multiple opinions. You either have to believe in sex addiction or not in this climate. There is no in-between. Both sides generally cling to their comfort zones, which creates an echo chamber that holds our field back from making progress on this issue.

Fear of Radical Religious Agendas and the Social Issues Surrounding Sex Addiction and Sexuality

As a label, sexual addiction has a reputation of being connected to religious conservatism. Many of the clients who come in for sexual addiction treatment also come from religious, conservative backgrounds. There are sex addiction therapists who have marketed religion. Some of these therapists have pushed their views onto their clients. Those advocating for sexual progress can view this marketing as a threat.

However, this reputation has led to schemas, suspicion, and stereotypes. I've been guilty of over-associating stereotypes with religious therapists myself. Based on my own experience and personal growth, let me say this. If you judge all therapists who are affiliated with a religion as sexually repressive, you're wrong. All communities are made up of a variety of perspectives on the topic of sexuality. As I've gotten to know therapists who integrate religious preferences into their practices, I know that this can be a resource for some clients. What separates harmful religious therapists from those who don't harm clients? Boundaries. When therapists have solid, personal boundaries, they know the limits of their responsibilities in sessions, and they avoid projecting their views of morality onto their clients.

With that said, there are also evangelical therapists and Christian counselors who treat sexual addiction and do so in a harmful manner. These professionals often label various sexual orientations, gender expressions, and sexual expressions as addictive. Some of these therapists have been CSAT trained, but evangelism isn't a part of the CSAT training process. In fact, the vast majority of extreme evangelical therapists aren't CSAT credentialed.

Although several Christian counselors treat sexual addiction, these counselors aren't all the same and there are those who are rigidly evangelical, and there are those who are more liberal. I don't practice Christian counseling myself, but I have peers who offer such services. For those looking for someone to help them process their Christian-based beliefs, these professionals can be a great asset. These counselors recognize and respect client boundaries without projecting their belief systems onto them. At the same time, they can offer insight into Christianity when it's an important part of the client's process.

Unfortunately, there are also evangelical therapists who have done the opposite. They believe that all of their clients must have goals that conform to the therapist's definition of Christianity. They use their license as a platform to advocate for their religious ideology, and they view their religious belief systems as superior. Using a therapeutic platform in this way can be shaming to clients who are already struggling with sexual or gender self-acceptance and authenticity.

Christianity isn't the only religious preference that can impact sexual and gender identity. However, in my experience, it's the most common religious background that fuels the controversy surrounding sex addiction. This is because SOCE is highly correlated with Christian evangelism. In therapy, the extreme religious views of a therapist can ignorantly shame clients. In those situations, therapists decide what is good and bad, and/or healthy and unhealthy for their clients.

Some research has shown correlations between religious shame and sexual compulsivity. In my experience of working with people with traumatic backgrounds, evangelism often leads to religious abuse. I've worked with countless clients who were taught to view their sexual desire as something that is dangerous and shameful. As therapists who help these clients, we have to appreciate sexuality and gender differences. We also have to understand our belief systems as well.

Our current political climate on LGBTQ rights further increases the sensitivity of discussions about religion in psychotherapy. Despite social advances for gay and lesbian individuals, religious arguments advocating against LGBTQ people continue to take their toll. So-called "religious freedom" and "bathroom" bills are shaming to LGBTQ individuals and couples. Current political platforms make it challenging to know whom to trust in religious conversations about therapy.

Although it's becoming increasingly rare, there are still several therapists who are part of the anti-LGBTQ movement. Some professionals believe that homosexuality is a curable and treatable "behavior problem." Anti-LGBTQ therapy groups use the term *sexual addiction* when describing homosexuality and gender variances. This is a hijacking of the term.

Twelve Step groups for sex addiction also add to the concerns about evangelism in sex addiction therapy. While most Twelve Step groups are friendly towards LGBTQ people, there are others that aren't. Many of those groups that are friendly to the LGBTQ community are still likely to stigmatize other relationship styles and sexual expression such as kink and polyamory.

Even worse, some churches offer Twelve Step groups that label homosexuality as "same-sex attraction" and treat it as a behavioral or addiction problem. Some of these churches even excommunicate their LGBTQ members until they conform and repress their sexual orientation or gender. These groups also advocate against healthy sexual behavior such as masturbation, while they also stigmatize sexual fantasy.

Religious evangelism has an undeniable influence on the clients who work with us in therapy. Sex and religion can have a complicated relationship. It's impossible to have an open dialogue about sex addiction without considering the influence of religion on the topic. Like most discussions that include morality and religion, these discussions often get intense.

Advocacy and Faux-Advocacy

As a long-term social progressive, it's important to me that the groups discussed in this book are advocated for. I understand and believe in the value of advocacy. However, there is something called *faux-advocacy* in our field that must be addressed. In these situations, professionals are using a social concern for themselves, rather than for a social cause. I've witnessed proponents on both sides of the argument on sex addiction use marginalized groups to advance their perspectives, gain attention, dominate, and ostracize others. These debates are used to incriminate therapists who hold different opinions. In the most heated exchanges, members who represent these groups are usually talked over and ignored. This isn't advocacy.

Of course, it's important to be an ally of marginalized groups; however, if you speak for a group without listening to representatives of that group, you're not advocating at all. You're actually doing more harm by using that group to promote your agenda. In every marginalized group, there are different people who hold different opinions on various topics. This includes the topic of sex addiction.

It's important to recognize the difference between isolated social discussions and advocacy. Isolation can lead to an echo chamber, which promotes stereotyping of other groups. Whereas open dialogue and personal responsibility are catalysts for true social change. It's difficult to learn more about people who disagree with you, but we have to step outside of our comfort zones to help our field improve and to socially progress.

Social change is also reliant upon everyone taking personal responsibility for their beliefs and behaviors and being mindful about their part in sociocultural problems. Everyone plays a role in the mistreatment of vulnerable groups. Hanging out in echo chambers keeps the foundations of mistreatment intact. Isolation encourages people to point fingers, make assumptions, and judge and criticize others. It also discourages people from taking personal responsibility for their part of the social system.

The sex addiction controversy is full of faux advocacy. There are a lot of professionals who are using social justice issues to attack the sex addiction label. These battles are often abandoned as soon as a debate about sex addiction is felt to have been won. This isn't about the advocacy of vulnerable groups at all. Instead, these groups are just being used to fight battles about sex addiction.

Faux advocacy such as this makes it more difficult for vulnerable groups to make progress. Their important messages get drowned out by political agendas of other people. These agendas can also lower the tolerance of peoples' ability to listen to the stories that really matter.

True advocacy is important. Identifying social concerns and discovering ways to best treat people is critical in the advancement of our field. This requires that we listen to some level of criticism, while also avoiding oversimplification of concerns. For example, I firmly believe that professionals who use evangelism to shame their clients should be held accountable. I also feel it's important to regularly critique labels and treatment approaches as a field. At the same time, the importance of the controversy over sex addiction transcends sex addiction itself. There are so many elements to this discussion. When the discussion is oversimplified, it ignores complex considerations of culture. Whereas when we make room for an open dialogue, our field can grow. However, these discussions also lead the way for broader social/cultural changes. After all, we're looked to as experts about people. This comes with an enormous responsibility.

Old Wounds and What We Have Learned the Hard Way

I've already discussed how religious evangelism impacts the sex addiction controversy. I also believe that some of the negative responses to sex addiction come from old wounds from the field of psychology. Psychology and sexuality have a complicated relationship. Like most fields, psychology has had a long learning curve. When it comes to sexuality, our field continues to be moving along this curve. Some would say that we've made progress, but gender and other consensual sexual behaviors are still included in the DSM as pathologized diagnoses.

This journey doesn't only reflect the current progression towards sexual positivity. There is a long, shameful background regarding sexuality that psychology itself has to own. One of the most shameful parts of this history includes the mistreatment of LGBTQ individuals. The shame from this era makes it difficult for sexually marginalized groups to trust therapists.

As late as 1973, homosexuality was still considered a valid mental health diagnosis. This wasn't completely removed from the DSM until 1987. The fourth version of the DSM continued to consider gender identity issues as a valid mental health diagnosis until 2014. Even now, the DSM-5 still includes a diagnosis for "gender dysphoria." Although this is reported to be a more politically correct term, dysphoria remains in a manual that is primarily intended for mental health diagnosis.

Issues surrounding sexual orientation and gender continue to this day. State and federal battles against SOCE continue. Most states continue to allow these practices. In fact, some state governments even advocate for them. There are still prominent members of the psychological and mental health fields who continue to insist that sexual orientation and gender are changeable.

LGBTQ competency is an ongoing issue in social work, marriage and family therapy, psychology, and counseling. Heterosexism and cisgender bias persist without the awareness of many therapists. These concepts are increasingly becoming recognized, appreciated and understood. However, there are many who don't recognize their bias, which can cause harm to their clients.

I would argue that there is even less competency regarding kink, BDSM, and non-monogamy. Our field continues to struggle with nonjudgment. Advocates point out that this can lead to ongoing labeling and shame. Bias can lead therapists to use a sex addiction label for these consensual expressions of sexuality.

Psychology has historical wounds surrounding the treatment of women and non-white groups as well. For example, the DSM has a long history of gender bias. This is especially true of personality disorders, but this isn't the only diagnostic group that is biased. To this day, there are several other diagnoses that are considered controversial.

These biases aren't new either. Many of the founders of the field of psychology are considered to be sexist by more modern scholars. Their perspectives on mental illness in women were likely misinterpretations of normal expressions of emotion. The labels placed on them failed to take larger social contexts into account.

Biases can marginalize racial and ethnic groups as well. Individuals from racial minorities can be unfairly and inaccurately labeled. Psychological research has primarily focused on perspectives that represent white perceptions and needs in therapy. Most approaches and interventions that have been developed normalize a white, heterosexual viewpoint, which can leave non-dominant groups feeling misinterpreted, judged, and even shamed in therapy.

Cultural awareness is important when providing sex-positive therapy to anyone who is dealing with sexually compulsive behavior. There are cultural influences that impact how members of different groups contend with emotions, trauma, and sexuality. For example, men and women view sex differently. Different groups have different experiences with emotional pain as it relates to sexuality.

As professionals, this means that we have a lot to balance when discussing sex. We have our own beliefs. We also have research to consider, but a lot of the research is biased in some way. As you have read, we also have a long history of pain inflicted on various groups relating to sexuality, mental health, and labels. Therefore, these topics get tense and awkward to discuss.

All people struggle with shame when identifying their biases. Therapists aren't immune to this. However, it's uncomfortable to accept these biases. Professionals, and the organizations who represent us, are faced with uncomfortable, but important responsibilities. We need to encourage open discussions about heterosexism, transphobia, sexual bias, racism, and sexism. People tend to avoid these discussions because they're often uncomfortable. Organizations also tend to discourage them to prevent dialogue that gets out of control. The problem with this is that over-censoring doesn't give professionals a way of processing sensitive, cultural information.

It can be overwhelming to identify everything that needs to change in our field. It's important to note that we can be change agents in these organizations. To do this, we have to identify our values. It also means we have to contend with our biases. Throughout this book, I will be naming some of the biases that are common. I encourage you to identify your values, but I also want you to look at biases and determine which ones apply to you. This is a daily practice. I call it a practice because some days we're better at healing than others. I've often failed at being open to perspectives that are different from my own and I know I will fail again. You will fail too if you're trying to be an agent of change. It's important to keep this in mind and circle back when you can.

Sex Addiction Therapy Research

Research—and the lack of it—causes some of the most intense debates on the subject of sex addiction. Critics of sexual addiction cite research providing evidence that it doesn't exist. On the other hand, those who are proponents of sex addiction treatment will point to research that "proves" its existence. In this debate, both sides of this argument often emphasize neurological research of brain responses to various sexual stimuli.

Some sexuality researchers argue that within brain imaging studies there is evidence that the brain responds in a particular way to sexual imagery and stimuli. The majority of this research focuses on pornography. Though, critics have cited issues with some of these studies. For example, some of the research is based on very small samples. Also, some of the images in these studies aren't conclusive in their representation of an addiction. Ongoing research needs to be conducted to further determine the validity of brain imagery as evidence supporting the existence of sex addiction.

Other researchers have utilized brain imagery in their studies supporting the theory that the opposite might be true. They offer evidence of brain imagery showing that there is no evidence of sexual addiction at all. In these studies, the imagery points away from addiction theories. Critics of this have argued that this research is biased.

Research is important, and it can help enhance our understanding of our work and our clients' problems. However, we also have to accept that research is limited in its applicability to actual therapy sessions. Psychology has long attempted to become more like medicine and "prescribe" treatment to specific conditions. However, there are also several critics who claim that the medicalization of our field has increased the mindlessness of therapists. These critics also claim that this encourages therapists to ignore relationships between emotional, spiritual, social, and cultural factors.

There is a lot of bias that goes into research as well. Obviously, there are several researchers who control for their own assumptions and bias. Several others take their preconceived notions into their studies and set them up so that they can prove their hypotheses to be true.

In general, I read the most extreme and bold statements that come from research with skepticism. When I read headlines such as "One study proved [insert any outcome]," I immediately ask myself, "What other possibilities could have led to this outcome?" I don't only do this with psychological research, but all studies. Research studies really are only puzzle pieces added to a puzzle. If one study claims to complete the entire puzzle, it's best to keep looking for missing pieces. Good research accepts that it's only a piece and not the entire picture.

Funding also plays a major role in research. The trends in how studies are funded discourage failures, which encourages the bias that I just discussed. There are also trends in research funding. Studies that follow these trends are more likely to get funded, while research that doesn't follow these trends is more likely to go ignored. Finally, researchers are often constrained for time, which can prevent them from asking tougher deeper questions.

Very few psychotherapy and sex therapy approaches have been extensively researched. Our field is loaded with information that hasn't been well-researched. In fact, many of our psychology and counseling students are still taught theory that has little research to back it up. Furthermore, there is a growing body of evidence that shows it's actually the therapeutic relationship that is more important than the actual approach that is utilized.

This doesn't mean that identifying evidenced-based approaches is useless. In fact, these approaches have helped many people. It also doesn't mean that we shouldn't do research or use it to better understand ways of helping people. We have to support our researchers. They help us fine-tune our field, identify new possibilities, and answer important questions. They also hold us accountable, while bringing increased credibility to our field.

When discussing controversial topics such as sex addiction, we need to have a balanced conversation about the vague, complicated elements of our field. Psychotherapy is difficult to research because we're dealing with the complexities of people. Therapy is largely an art. It requires creativity and self-awareness in the practitioner. It also involves the nuances of therapeutic relationship factors such as transference, countertransference, and resonance. When people get into the debate on sex addiction, these factors are often ignored by all sides.

Most intense debates on controversial topics are more complex than "either/or" classifications. The truth tends to exist somewhere in the middle. Although research is important in better understanding our clients' issues, our clients' perspectives about their own problems matter as well. There are broad considerations in our clients' lives. Therefore, I believe that helping people with sexual compulsivity is much more complex than proving its existence or non-existence.

The goal of research shouldn't be to prove anything. Research simply provides a groundwork for future studies. For example, we have to be cautious about using a brain disease model when discussing sex addiction problems. Some studies suggest that this could be a possibility, while others indicate that it isn't as well. In other words, our field needs to follow research so that new questions can be asked until a consensus is reached.

Evidence-Based Treatment and Label Confusion

All addictions can be difficult to define. Process addictions can be even more difficult to define. The definition of sex addiction is often broad and misunderstood. Is it too much sex? Is it cheating? Is it perpetration? These are common misconceptions about the definition of sex addiction, which often lead to concerns from critics that sex addiction therapy can be void of evidence-based treatment interventions.

I want to use another process addiction to demonstrate the complexities of addiction labels. The DSM-5 includes the Gambling Disorder diagnosis under its category of addictive disorders. The research is early and inconclusive whether physiological symptoms would represent addiction. Physical symptoms of tolerance and withdrawal are challenging to assess in non-substance abuse, compulsive behaviors. Even still, process addiction experts have identified physical withdrawal and tolerance symptoms that occur in process addictions.

In the DSM-IV era, addiction terminology was linked to the diagnosis of dependence. This diagnosis had the possibility of being given with or without physiological symptoms. The non-physiological symptoms of this diagnosis included unsuccessful efforts to stop using the substance, time being consumed by the substance use, and giving up other important activities for the substance. Therefore, people could be diagnosed as "dependent" without physiological symptoms.

The DSM-5 changed its criteria, but only to further encompass both abuse and dependence symptoms. In fact, the DSM identified these symptoms as "addictive," rather than calling it "dependence." Dependence terminology isn't used at all in the DSM-IV. The non-physiological symptoms of these addictive disorders are still listed in the current criteria for substance-related addictions.

DSM Limitations in Finding the Right Label

We have to be realistic when utilizing the DSM to back up discussions surrounding addiction terminology. It's unfair to pretend that the DSM is a perfect document that is based only on research and evidence. The DSM-5 was criticized for its lack of evidence to support many of the diagnoses within it.

At the same time, concerns regarding diagnoses outside of the DSM are legitimate. Without a standardized process, mental health professionals can be given too much freedom in diagnosing. Professionals can pathologize normal variances in human behavior. Rather than identifying and addressing issues that need legitimate help, anything outside cultural norms can be treated as a mental health problem. This has already happened in our history both inside and outside the field of psychology.

Many of the diagnoses within the DSM-5 are controversial. It can be difficult to divide the lines between "disordered" and "variable." This also becomes increasingly difficult with issues relating to sex and gender. Sexuality has a long history of having norms tied to it. Since the beginning of written history, there is evidence that all cultures and civilizations had norms associated with sex. The DSM struggles to draw distinct differences between unhealthy symptoms and consensual sex and gender expression.

Diagnosing people purely for variances in arousal, gender, and expression is sex negative. Some "fetishistic" diagnoses are consensual variances in human sexuality, yet are still included in the DSM. On the other hand, sex positivity regards variations in sexual behavior as appropriate and healthy.

Physiological and neurological symptoms are important considerations when defining an addiction. This is true of sex addiction as well; yet, these aren't the only symptoms that would need consideration. As you're well aware, there are social and family consequences that we work with on a regular basis. These consequences can't go ignored when conceptualizing and defining an addiction.

Whichever way you look at the definition, it's controversial. In sex addiction cases, the symptoms described by most people highly correlate with symptoms of people living with other addictive disorders. The consequences similarly correlate as well. Whether it's the relational, social, or emotional impact of the behavior, the outcomes can be very similar.

This isn't to say that these factors alone mean that "addiction" is the best label for the problem. At the same time, it's understandable why clients, clinicians, and researchers have identified these behavioral outcomes as an addiction. Up to this point, solid, neurobiological evidence of addiction in sexual behavior has yet to be clearly identified. Until that day, ongoing controversies on this topic will persist.

The most important part of our work is to help our clients. In my experience, they'll identify with a label that they feel best fits. Some will not identify with any label at all.

Finding Evidenced-Based Treatment for Sex Addiction

An argument against sex addiction therapy that I've heard many times is that an "addiction model" can't be used to help with sexual compulsivity. I've always been confused about the meaning of this argument. As a therapist who has worked with addictions for many years, I'm aware that standard addiction treatment includes relapse prevention, solution-focused treatment, identification of triggers, in-depth trauma work, and mindfulness-based cognitive behavioral therapy. In general, several of these therapeutic approaches have been shown to be effective in treating various mood and behavioral problems, as well as addiction issues.

Client involvement is also an important consideration when searching for an evidenced-based approach to treat sex addiction. Clients hold a lot of responsibility in their therapeutic process. Arguably, outcomes would improve if clinicians could *make* clients engage in the process. The outcomes would also improve if there was a linear progression that moved clients from problematic symptoms to success. Unfortunately, the process for clients is rarely, if ever linear.

The role of the therapist is to offer what is needed, but clients are responsible for identifying their problems. Some might need specific tools. Some need crisis management and advice. Others need validation and space to work through their situations. Clients are often unclear of what they need out of the therapy process. Therapists have a critical role in helping clients sort out what is most needed in each case. Therefore, they progress at different rates and some don't progress at all. When measuring the outcomes of a particular approach, it's difficult for research to consider all of these dynamics.

It's also important to remember that no two clients are the same. A certain combination of interventions and approaches might work for one client while failing with another. No particular approach or form of support should be blamed for this. Instead, we have to work together to understand what makes particular interventions work for some and fail for others. Flexibility in interventions can help us best serve our clients. In the end, we have to base our work on how clients respond and the goals that they've set.

Balancing the Importance of the Twelve Steps in Sexual Compulsivity

In my experience, when professionals argue against the "addiction model," it seems like they're arguing against two primary things. One argument is against labeling sexual behavior patterns as an addiction. The other is against the utilization of a "Twelve Step Model" in the treatment of sexually compulsive behavior. We've already discussed issues with labeling at length. It's important to talk about the Twelve Steps as well, because they're part of the controversy surrounding sex addiction.

Addictions are often treated by utilizing the Twelve Steps as a treatment approach by addiction programs and therapists. When people argue against "the addiction model," I believe that this is often what they're referring to. I've had clients who were living with sexual compulsivity who greatly benefited from Twelve Step support groups. I've also had other clients who've found little to no benefit from them. I know that I may upset some people by saying this, but I've also seen Twelve Step groups harm some of my clients and even some of my friends.

Before we get into balancing the discussion about the Twelve Steps, I want to be transparent. I am not a Twelve Step therapist. I never have been; however, I've had many clients who have benefited from them. I've found it beneficial for these clients to do "meaning work" in their groups. In this type of work, they can identify benefits from participating in these groups. Deepening this understanding can be quite empowering for clients because it brings meaning to their recovery.

The Twelve Steps and the CSAT Credential

The Twelve Steps are a source of regular criticism of the CSAT training and the credential itself. The CSAT credential utilizes workbooks, assessments and exercises that were created by Dr. Patrick Carnes and other well-known CSAT therapists. Two popular books, *Facing the Shadows* and *Recovery Zone*, include many of the activities that are shared in these trainings. These books have some elements of the Twelve Steps in them. There are also other elements of interpersonal work included.

It's unfair to place The Twelve Steps as an antagonist to psychotherapy, which has been done in several debates about sex addiction. The Steps often overlap with common therapeutic interventions. For example, "Step One" could be interpreted as identifying with acceptance of a problem that you have. This would also align with a motivational interviewing process, which is widely accepted as a recommended way of working with compulsive behavior.

CSAT training materials also focus on some elements of cognitive-behavioral theory, as well as attachment theory. I'm not discussing these materials because I believe they're the only activities that help clients. At the same time, we need to be fair and factual when criticizing an approach. These materials benefit some clients, while others would prefer alternative approaches. Like most things, the best methods aren't going to be dictated by the therapy community. They're going to be dictated by what helps the person sitting with you in a therapy session.

Religion is one factor that makes the Twelve Steps controversial. As I've previously stated, the Twelve Steps emphasize the importance of "God." Although this may be helpful for some, there are others who will not want this in their lives or as part of their treatment. Clinicians have a duty to respect this. Unfortunately, I've seen this line crossed multiple times by therapists. It's important to point out that CSAT therapists aren't the only ones who have crossed this boundary. All therapists have a responsibility to respect their clients' boundaries, rather than preach to them.

We also have to recognize situations that can be shameful and harmful to our clients and work to change them. Many religious groups and therapists who practice SOCE have encouraged clients to attend Twelve Step support groups that promote shame. As sexual health professionals, we need to understand the obvious and subtle impact that different organizations have on our clients. This can help them develop lasting support networks.

Defining "Healthy" Sexuality

When it comes to sex addiction, the most well recognized Twelve Step groups include Sexaholics Anonymous (SA), Sex Addicts Anonymous (SAA) and Sex and Love Addicts Anonymous (SLAA). These are just a few of the organizations that utilize Twelve Step support.

There are support groups for partners of those with sexually compulsive behavior as well. Groups such as Codependents of Sex Addicts (COSA) focus on offering Twelve Step support to partners of sex addicts. This is similar to –ANON groups offered to family and friends of those with drug and alcohol problems. These groups offer support in a majority of cities across the country every day.

Although these groups can offer great support to our clients, we need to know where we're referring them. Twelve Step support groups have different group values. Our clients can be shamed by these values if we're not careful. Therefore, it's important to gain an understanding of the values systems of these groups. It's also important to regularly check in with clients to determine their interpretations of these values. Therapists can process problems with clients as they arise.

SA, in particular, has been the focus of major debates about sex addiction. SA has a definition of "healthy" sexuality, which can be shaming to all of the vulnerable groups discussed in this book. This organization defines healthy sexual experiences as those that occur between a man and a woman. For people who are single, the SA belief is that they should abstain from sex altogether.

Obviously, as a gay male, I have issues with an organizational definition of healthy sex being only between a man and a woman. I also don't believe that all—or even most—people should abstain from masturbation. Masturbation is a normal part of human sexuality and development. I believe that advocating for an anti-masturbation society is unrealistic and shaming.

I also have concerns about this definition of healthy sexuality when it comes to adolescent development. Adolescents can be vulnerable to a label of sex addiction for their normal expressions of sexual behavior. Some parents may panic when they notice their child is masturbating. Definitions such as the SA definition of healthy sexuality have the potential to encourage over-labeling of sex addiction. This can cause adolescents to go through "treatment" for something that isn't a problem at all.

Apart from SA, Celebrate Recovery is another Twelve Step group that has been shaming of the LGBTQ community. It encourages LGBTQ people to assimilate their sexual orientation and gender to heterosexuality and cis-genderism. This perspective is based on religious evangelism and is considered harmful and unethical. Sadly, many churches refer people to such organizations. This makes the coming out process a long and detrimental road for LGBTQ youth and adults.

How do we have grounded discussions about sex addiction with these harmful groups out there? Each day, I'm hopeful we'll inch closer to a society that appreciates all genders and orientations. At the same time, I know I can't personally erase SA and Celebrate Recovery from the map.

I have to remind myself that SA and Celebrate Recovery's definitions and organizational value systems reflect cultural and social issues that are larger than sex addiction. Several cultural, religious, and social constructs encourage sexual and gender shame. I focus on where I can be a change agent, while reminding myself that change doesn't happen overnight. This can be sad, frustrating, and exhausting. Sometimes, I really do well with this, and other times it's more difficult to stay focused.

I also appreciate the fact that being a therapist and sexuality professional puts me in an important position. Clients often come to me for help with navigating through their journeys. Traveling with them through their life journeys has helped me stay grounded and

> balanced. What would you say helps you stay grounded and balanced with these cultural struggles?

The Twelve Steps aren't only utilized in support groups. They're often considered a form of treatment. Critics of sex addiction are often strongly opposed to the use of the Twelve Steps as a treatment approach. There is some legitimacy for the basis of these concerns because there is limited evidence showing positive outcomes when the Twelve Steps are used as the backbone of therapy.

To help our field progress on this topic, we have to have fair discussions. When considering criticism about Twelve Step treatment approaches, we can't ignore the reality of addiction treatment in general. There isn't much that has been proven to be extremely effective in the treatment of any addiction. Even the most effective treatment approaches demonstrate poor overall outcomes.

Finally, we also have to accept another bias about the Twelve Steps that can increase the divide. I've heard of many situations where colleagues and friends were shamed by other therapists for not utilizing the Twelve Steps in therapy. It's important to accept and appreciate different approaches, creativity, and talent. Mistreatment of our colleagues promotes division and defensiveness. Research shows that eclecticism is most useful in treating mental health issues and addictions. Empathy is another critical element of psychotherapy. There isn't one linear way of empathizing with someone. Therefore, those who utilize other approaches should be welcomed, rather than scrutinized, belittled or judged.

Ending the Rumor Mill

Sadly, I've heard several rumors about both CST and CSAT credential processes. One of the most damaging rumors is that IITAP trains its therapists to use SOCE. As a gay male who has sat through the entire CSAT process, this is simply untrue.

Slander has extended far and wide between these communities of therapists and within them as well. There are bystanders who allow the rumors to exist. There are also hostile perpetrators of these rumors who turn their rage onto anyone who tries to correct them. As terrifying as it is, these people are mental health "professionals."

I've also heard rumors regarding the CST credential and AASECT trainings from many CSAT therapists. To help our clients, we have to stop encouraging baseless rumors. If you hear something that you're unsure about, go to the source. Get more information.

If you spread rumors, you're hurting your colleagues and hurting our field as well. In fact, rumors can even prevent clients from seeking out the help of a therapist who could support them. In this book, I will be discussing the harm of twisting and bending a social cause to fit the needs of your personal agenda. At this point in this book, I want to remind everyone how rumors and slander are harmful to our field. Even worse, they encourage societal hierarchies that end up harming minority groups. Be the professional who calls out BS, rather than one who promotes it.

Evidence-Based Illusions

The issues surrounding evidence-based practices aren't only related to the treatment of sex addiction. This movement is one that is pushed throughout the entire field of psychotherapy. On paper, being "evidenced-based" sounds nice; however, there are many complicated elements to therapeutic effectiveness that are difficult to measure.

Therapists also regularly and wrongly assume that their approaches to therapy are evidenced-based. Some of the most valued approaches in our field aren't evidence-based at all. This doesn't mean that there is no value in them. Therapists will often assume that their approaches are based in solid research when they see improvements in their clients. We have to recognize how limited the research is at this time.

In research, correlation isn't always causation. When there are positive outcomes, it's unclear whether these results are coming from the therapeutic approach or from other factors. It's well-known that therapeutic relationships are often more important than the treatment modality used with clients. Outcomes may be related to the treatment approach. Still, the therapeutic process may be more about the alliance with the client than the actual approach that is utilized by the practitioner.

When assessing the evidence of the outcomes of particular treatment modalities, it's easier to assess short-term approaches. Long-term benefits can be difficult to measure due to dwindling numbers within samples. There is limited research on some highly regarded "evidenced-based" approaches that have led to questions about the long-term benefits of short-term therapy. For example, there was a time when Brief Solution Focused Therapies (BSFT) gained so much popularity because research reported on its positive outcomes. To add to this, it was cost-effective. At the time, clinicians found this approach to be simple to implement and utilize.

As years passed, clinicians began to report that some of their clients who had previously shown improvements had re-entered therapy. A significant number of them were also worse off than when they first entered treatment. I'm not suggesting that the interventions used in BSFT caused a more severe relapse. Clients often initially benefit from easy-to-apply and simple-to-understand interventions. Though, this can leave deeper issues unaddressed.

Again, we need to research and understand as much as we can about the varying treatment options we offer our clients. We also have to acknowledge that approaches described as evidence-based aren't always the best. Individual clients require individualized treatment. Evidence-based treatment has been used as a way of standardizing care for clients in medicine and mental health. Although this has helped make healthcare more efficient in some situations, it also leaves several clients falling through the cracks.

Beyond Labels and Moving Forward

The sex addiction label has been misused by many therapists. We all have to acknowledge this to bridge the divide on sex addiction. Unfortunately, there are a lot of evangelical groups that continue to view sexuality through a heteronormative, traditional perspective. Although sex addiction therapy itself isn't based in evangelism, we have to take time to distance ourselves from those who use therapy as a way to project their views and values onto others. We can't address a problem if we don't accept that it exists, and call it out when it occurs.

Sexual addiction labels must be handled with care when therapists work with clients who are interested in nontraditional relationships, gender, and sexual expression. Therapy should offer a safe place for clients to sort out their desire, expression, and arousal. Providing such a place will be further discussed later in this book.

Outcomes are important. Debates among clinicians are essential. Therapists need to incorporate clients' perspectives in their research, too. I believe that some arguments take attention away from clients' needs and their points of view.

When the dust settles, there may be substantial evidence that demonstrates that addiction terminology always hinders client progress. At this time, such solid evidence doesn't exist. Obviously, there are times when clients will use the label as a response to cultural shame. I will be discussing how to handle these situations in a way that promotes authenticity throughout this book without invalidating your clients in the process.

A Label Made for the Greedy?

One of the most condemning arguments against sex addiction treatment is that the label of sex addiction was created because of greed. Critics of sex addiction often claim that this is a fictitious problem created only to make money for therapists and treatment centers. There are some valid points made about the addiction industry as a whole. I've also seen this argument turn into far-reaching nonsense as well.

The Culture of Financial Shame in Helping Professions

Our society has strong beliefs towards financial gain in psychotherapy, counseling, and social work. As the owner of a group practice and a counselor supervisor, I know that helping professionals are usually humble folks. We struggle to own our goals. We can also struggle to own our worthiness of making a living.

We work in what is called a "giving profession." In this field, one of the most insulting criticisms a therapist can get is to be labeled as someone who "wants to make money." These undertones can be heard in our education, but they also extend further out into our culture and workplaces. Our overall societal undertone is that human service workers aren't financially worth much at all.

Over the years, I've seen a lot of therapists practically give their services away for free. And yes, many of them are CSATs. These professionals are hardly the most vocal voices in our field, but many of them are just as talented—if not more so. Yet, they feel guilty about earning money.

This financial shame expands outward into our culture. Insurance companies underpay the time and effort dedicated to our clients. Public programs do the same by paying very little to therapists who work with the highest needs. Meanwhile, therapists offer some of the most intense and consistent one-on-one time in the health industry.

It's unreasonable to shame therapists for wanting to make a profit. In a capitalistic society, we decide for ourselves what we want out of our careers. There's nothing wrong with doing what we love, helping others, and making a profitable living at the same time. These things don't have to be mutually exclusive.

Some professionals enjoy appreciation and notoriety. Others want to help those who can't afford therapy services. There are those who want to make bigger social changes. Identifying your own goals is a gift, not a personal and professional flaw. When we create a space where therapists are able to establish goals without being shamed for them, we can better serve our clients.

Obviously, it wouldn't be okay to create a problem just to make a profit. However, unfair accusations of greed do nothing to identify the real culprits. In mental health, like medicine, we have to know where acceptable profitability transforms into greed. I've worked with more therapists who are afraid of making money than therapists who are "greedy." I also don't believe that therapists are greedy when they set financial goals.

When Consumerism Becomes Greed in Addiction Treatment

It's sad to say, but I have seen profitability eclipse ethics in treatment. In addiction treatment, I've observed one line violated more than any other. There are several programs who disregard their ethical responsibility to only admit clients to the least restrictive level of care, just so they can fill empty beds. In general, clients should only be encouraged to participate in the least restrictive setting for their problem. I know there are clients who make a choice to participate in residential programs because they want to engage in an intense level of care to learn and grow. This isn't what I'm talking about here. I'm calling out how inappropriate it is for addiction treatment programs to inflate clients' problems so they can get them into their program. This, unfortunately, happens often.

The American Society of Addiction Medicine (ASAM) has developed levels of addiction treatment, but these levels of care aren't always respected. The ASAM levels range from simple amounts of education to complete hospitalization. I've worked with a lot of people who have benefited from Intensive Outpatient Programs (IOPs), residential programs, and hospitalizations. It's true—these programs can help people. At the same time, I've also seen clients enter addiction programs without an addiction problem at all.

Hospitals, long-term care, and residential settings have enormous pressure to bring in large amounts of money to sustain their profitability. However, the overwhelming need to pay for overhead costs, while making a profit, increases the pressure to keep beds filled. Some of these places use unethical admission and discharge processes to make money.

I've seen this in the sex addiction field as well. Although many programs practice ethics in their admission and discharge practices, there are some that lack such integrity. This is a serious problem in medicine and mental health that goes way beyond sexual addiction, but the sex addiction field needs to contend with it just the same. The treatment of non-addictive behavior in addiction treatment facilities taints the entire field. It also contributes to driving up of medical costs, which further limits resources.

I don't know what the solution is to this problem. However, if we're having a balanced discussion on sexual compulsivity, acknowledgment is critical. We can't pretend that this issue doesn't exist at all.

Working Towards Balance in Perspectives

Entire books have been written about the controversy over sex addiction. For the purposes of this book, I wanted to draw some basic awareness to the controversies. I hope this helps you find a mindful and balanced mind-space when working with clients and talking with colleagues.

Almost all professionals encounter clients who are living with compulsive sexual behavior. I encourage you to engage in multiple trainings and programs. You can learn about different perspectives and theories and identify various ways of integrating these approaches. This takes effort and commitment. It requires that you discover what is most authentic to you, so you can offer support to your clients. Most importantly, integrating approaches keeps clients at the center of the therapeutic process.

2

Identifying the Problem

When someone comes into therapy for a problem with sexual compulsivity, the case can become complicated. It's difficult to know where to turn for information and training. Opinions tend to be pretty split on this topic, which can make it confusing when you're trying to conceptualize a case. To add to this, clients come into our offices with a broad array of situations that require our help.

Before assessing your clients, it's important to understand your perspectives on sexuality. We all have judgments. We also have boundaries that we have established in our own relationships. Of course, our clients' boundaries are going to be different than our own; however, our boundaries impact our perceptions. In the psychotherapy field, there are differing perspectives about various sexual behaviors.

Before we get into a discussion on bias, it's essential for us to acknowledge that perceptions are a part of being human. Therapists shouldn't pretend they have no biases. At the same time, it can feel shameful to own up to them. We're going to discuss bias a lot throughout this book. I want you to start thinking about it now. When you take time to think about it, you can begin the process of mindful awareness when helping your clients.

Here are some common perceptions that can cause problems when conceptualizing a case:

- Pornography use is always wrong and unhealthy.
- Kink is a curable trauma re-enactment.
- Open relationships are immoral and impossible.
- Adolescent pornography use is always addictive.
- Men who are attracted to men are always gay.
- Pain with sexual play is unhealthy.
- People are either gay or straight.
- People should never fantasize or objectify others.
- Sex should only take place when there is love.
- Gender is assigned at birth.
- Relationships should only include two monogamous people.

There are several other misperceptions that aren't included in this list. Many of these issues are described in greater depth throughout this book. Again, the purpose of this list is to encourage you to identify perceptions that might already exist in your mind. Some of them you already recognize while you may not have noticed others prior to reading about them.

The Blurry Line of Addiction

If you're a concrete person, here's a warning. This book may frustrate you. I am going to name some standard definitions used by therapists to identify sex addiction in their clients; however, when we're working with the vulnerable groups in this book, there is no way to completely avoid vagueness.

The controversy surrounding sex addiction can lead to myths. A few of these myths include:

- The label of sex addiction always helps people in their therapeutic process.
- No one is ever a sex or porn addict.
- Vulnerable sexual and gender subgroups are never sex addicts.
- If your client identifies as a sex or porn addict, you need to correct them immediately.

I believe that you need to follow your client when using any diagnostic label. This is especially true of addiction labels. Your client will give you information about how they identify and what they're looking for from you. Validating and understanding their experiences is more critical to the process than any label you can assign them.

At the same time, you don't want your client to wander too far into any extremes. Clients may have rigid beliefs about their identity, sex, or their relationships. When they hang out in extreme thinking, they're at an increased risk of covering up their authentic identities with an addiction. There are gentle ways that therapists can confront this, which I will discuss throughout this book.

I'm also going to discuss some considerations that I want you to think about throughout this book. These considerations will transcend the importance of the sex addiction label because they focus on our clients' overall experiences. Respecting the broad narrative of our clients' lives can blur the defining lines of a sex addiction. If the most important thing for your client to figure out in therapy is whether they identify as an addict or not, then of course you're going to process that. In my experience, that is rare. The label itself is usually only one of several things that clients want to process during their time in therapy.

Three Critical Sexually Connective Elements

All client cases that relate to sexuality and relationships include three critical elements: honesty, self-acceptance, and consensual agreements. I assess these elements when I'm working with clients to monitor for interpersonal and sexual incongruence. Whether people are dealing with compulsive behavior or not, these elements can help therapists identify where clients need to go deeper into therapeutic work. When it comes to vulnerable groups, these elements are even more critical. Incongruence and a struggle with personal values are common among people who live outside of traditional sexual and gender norms.

Let me address each of these issues relating to sexual congruence.

1. Honesty.

Unfortunately, dishonesty is often a theme in sexuality. Sometimes, shame prevents people from being honest about their sexual desires in their relationships. This feeling can come from topics that are considered sexually taboo; however, it may also be related to an overall struggle with authenticity. This type of personal struggle can go well beyond sexuality and also reflects issues with relationship connection and vulnerability. Therapists need to help clients identify the sources of dishonesty so they can effectively address them.

Dishonesty and silence are threats to trust in relationships. Trust is a unifying force in any relationship. It's part of the foundation that holds people together in their relationships. When this foundation is fractured, relationships often fall apart.

Therapists need to look for compulsive levels of dishonesty when clients are dealing with sexual compulsivity. Dishonesty can include someone being dishonest with themselves, as well as chronically lying to other people. The authentic struggle of withholding information can become part of this compulsive process as well. When clients struggle with dishonesty, I know that they're also struggling with disconnection. Sexual disconnection is no exception to this.

2. Self-acceptance.

Self-acceptance can be challenging for people who belong to non-dominant groups in our society. Culturally, we have strict, even puritanical roots that continue to impact our ideas of sexuality and gender. Our cultural struggle with accepting variances in sexual orientation and gender is an example of our ongoing struggle with these roots. In sex-positive therapy, our goal is always to encourage clients to accept themselves for who they are as people.

Clinicians also need to be understanding and empathetic to the cultural processes that individuals go through. Race, ethnicity, religion, sexual orientation, and gender all impact self-acceptance. I'll discuss this in more detail later, but for now I want to point out that therapists often minimize these struggles. Therapists can help in this process, but they can hinder it as well.

We have to assess levels of self-acceptance when working with problems of sexual compulsivity. Therapists must help clients identify whether behavior patterns are reflective of a compartmentalized need for self-expression. We also have to be careful not to put clients into a framework of sexuality that doesn't fit their story.

3. Consensual agreements.

Therapists aren't the morality police for their clients. Clients come into therapy with complicated and messy situations. They might be confused or incongruent. This can become even messier when dealing with issues of relationships, passion, and sex.

Unfortunately, our culture has several expectations and assumptions about sex. These norms can prevent people from having honest and open communication in their relationships. Some of these norms are so powerful that they keep these interests suppressed. This can lead to hiding, withholding information, and outright lying. Much of our work, especially when working with vulnerable groups, involves helping our clients open lines of open communication. It also involves helping them reach relationship agreements.

In working with cases of sexual compulsivity, therapists have to remain aware that a lot of people will come in to therapy because they're confused about their problems. Some of these clients will not have a compulsive issue at all. At the same time, some of them may have feelings for someone outside of the primary relationship. They may have an interest in opening up the relationship. Or there might be a desire to engage in an activity that is new to the person or the relationship.

Sexual relationships obviously need to be consensual. Although this may sound like common sense, it can be complicated. For example, people define sex differently. It's also sometimes complicated to identify what should remain private within relationships. Therefore, we often have to help our clients establish these consensual agreements in therapy.

Assessment Concerns and Controversies

Not surprisingly, therapeutic assessments of sexual compulsivity have also been controversial. Critics of sex addiction therapy are often critical of the assessments and definitions that sexual addiction professionals utilize in their treatment. The following are common criticisms of these assessments: they're invalid, they pathologize non-normative sexual behavior, they're white-normative, and they're heteronormative.

Clinicians must be aware of cultural norms when conducting any assessment. This is no different when we use assessment tools to identify the problems associated with sexual compulsivity. Therapeutic tools require us to remain open to balanced criticism in order to improve. Also, all professionals have to utilize cultural competency when using any assessment tool.

Secrecy, values, and judgment are always involved with issues of sexuality. When assessing for sexual compulsivity, you must remain mindful of important and delicate factors. There are important assessment considerations for non-traditional relationships and non-heterosexual clients. If you're not cautious, you can mislabel consensual sexual behavior as problematic or even addictive.

Lesbian, gay, queer, and bisexual men and women can have a lot of shame surrounding their sexual orientation. When assessing for sexual compulsivity, you must be mindful when you're working with these clients as well. For example, meeting up for sex in public places is common in the personal histories of a lot of gay men. Historically, there haven't been very many safe places for gay men to meet up for sex. Therefore, it was common for them to explore their sexuality in these places. Some sexual compulsivity screening and assessment tools identify this type of behavior as problematic. These items must be considered through a culturally sensitive lens. Therapists have to identify whether the behavior is truly compulsive in nature. It's important to ask clarifying questions to avoid mislabeling this group.

Clinicians also have to remain aware of other mental health and addiction concerns. Clients who come into therapy for sexual addiction may be dealing with compulsivity that is secondary to another issue. Therefore, the assessment process must include ruling out depression and anxiety, as well as other issues. Some people resort to numbing behavior to cope with the emotions that they don't recognize and know how to manage.

Clinicians must also pay particular attention to rule out Bipolar Disorders and Attention Deficit and Hyperactivity Disorder (ADHD). Impulsivity is common for these two diagnoses. This impulsivity can be repetitive in nature, which can make it look like it is compulsive. Impulsivity can also lead to compulsivity when the outcome is one that is pleasurable and coping tools are missing.

Substance abuse and alcohol abuse issues should also be ruled out. Many people use substances to enhance a particular sexual experience. Some only engage in a specific behavior pattern when they're using the substance. In these situations, the primary issue has to be identified. I have found the following questions incredibly important to ask myself to further identify the most significant issues in my clients:

- Is substance abuse the central problem?
- Does the sexual compulsivity increase the likelihood of substance use?

- Does a sexual behavior need to be experienced with a substance in a compulsive way?

Finally, personality disorder traits, features, and diagnoses should also be assessed. This can help you identify whether you're dealing with someone who has the capacity to connect. This information will also assist you in making sense of patterns of attachment. These traits are critical to identifying issues with control and dependence in our clients' relationships.

The Sexual Addiction Label and Beyond

As you can see, assessing for a sex addiction can be very complicated. To correctly utilize a label, it's important to have a way of validating its appropriateness. The many layers of sexuality and social stigmas can make assessing clients for sex addiction complex. It's important for therapists to remind themselves that these complexities are often more relevant than the addiction label itself.

IITAP trains CSAT therapists to use the following criteria to identify sex addiction. As you will see, this is very similar to the DSM-IV criteria for substance dependence. A person must exhibit three or more of the following to be considered a sex addict by utilizing this criterion.

1. Recurrent failure (pattern) to resist sexual impulses to engage in specific sexual behaviors.
2. Engaged in sexual behaviors to a greater extent or over a more extended period than intended.
3. Long-standing desire, or a history of unsuccessful efforts to stop, reduce, or control sexual behaviors.

4. Spent excessive time obtaining sex, being sexual, or recovering from sexual experiences.
5. Obsessed with preparing for sexual activities.
6. Frequently engaged in sexual behavior when expected to be fulfilling occupational, academic, domestic, or social obligations.
7. Continued sexual behavior despite knowing it has caused or exacerbated social, financial, psychological, or physical problems.
8. Increased the intensity, frequency, number, or risk of sexual behaviors to achieve the desired effect, or experienced diminished effect when continuing behaviors at the same level of intensity, frequency, number, or risk.
9. Given up or limited social, occupational, or recreational activities because of sexual behavior.
10. Become upset, anxious, restless, or irritable if unable to engage in sexual behavior.

When is the Label Appropriate?

In my experience, diagnostic labels rarely help clients. I can hear people jeering me now. Let me explain. It's imperative to listen to our clients' problems and symptoms. With this information, we're likely to identify a diagnosis that seems appropriate for their situation. In all of my work with clients over the years, I've seen few situations where labels were the most beneficial aspect of therapy.

On the other hand, I've found it very useful to ask my clients what they think and feel about a particular label. This gives me information about how they're assessing the problem and identifying with it. Processing in this way has promoted ongoing dialogue about client perceptions of their issues.

In working with sex addiction, I've seen clients identify with this particular label. This identification has helped them understand past behaviors and has given them a framework that can help them make sense of their patterns of behavior. At the same time, I've worked with a lot of people who don't identify with the label at all. Rather than getting bogged down by a label, I've found that these clients do best when they have space and respect to identify their own problems.

When clients come to us for help, they're often in a crisis. Their relationship is in complete turmoil and they have little awareness of how they got into this situation. When the crisis includes relationship issues such as multiple affairs, clients more regularly suspect that they're dealing with sex addiction. This doesn't mean that the client is dealing with a sex addiction; however, some research is suggesting that people are relatively good at identifying their own problems. Therefore, it's worth investigating the labels that clients identify with.

When the label fits, it can help clients unpack a variety of other interpersonal issues. Those who come in for sex addiction therapy can struggle with emotional identification and compartmentalization. Working on emotions and past issues will be important in their future work. This label can be a foundational resource that sets a tone to discuss the importance and benefits of other deeper work.

When the label isn't forced onto clients, they may also find a sense of community by using it. Again, not all of my clients have benefited from the Twelve Steps. Those who do find these groups beneficial often cite shame reduction as one of the primary benefits of attending them. One of the hallmarks of shame is that you feel very alone. Hearing other peoples' stories can remind our clients that they aren't alone. Sharing their stories with an empathetic group can also help them regain a sense of self-worth.

When Doesn't the Label Work?

The sex addiction label can lower client involvement in therapy when it doesn't resonate with their experience. This is especially true of groups who are vulnerable of being wrongfully labeled, or who have a cultural history of sexual discrimination. In this book, we're going to talk about many of these groups, which include:

- Lesbian and gay individuals.
- Bisexual individuals.
- Those who identify as queer.
- Transgender and non-binary people.
- Those in polyamorous and open relationships.
- People with "fetishes."
- People who enjoy kink and BDSM.

Members of these groups sometimes feel very suspicious of the sex addiction label. It's critical to validate this suspicion. These feelings can come from experiences of shame related to their desires and needs for expression. Some of these clients have had abusive therapeutic relationships with a therapist who was shaming. Others have experienced cultural traumas surrounding their sexual orientation and gender. All of these things can teach these people that they need to be wary of therapists.

The sex addiction label can also be a problem for clients who use it as a way of shaming away their own authenticity. Unfortunately, there are many stigmas in our society that keep people from accepting who they are. Stigmas can be even more prevalent with sexuality and gender variances. I've worked with a lot of people who have assigned themselves with the sex addiction label in hopes that they'll conform and eradiate these variances.

Working with clients who have incorrectly self-diagnosed with a sex addiction can be challenging. Getting into a power struggle with these clients about the label is pointless and even harmful. Instead, I recommend that you work to gently focus on barriers to authenticity. Obviously, your clients will dictate how much of this they can tolerate. This can take a long time and requires a lot of patience. As time passes, you may be able to reflect on the self-prescribed label. It's so much more powerful when your clients rid themselves of an inappropriate label than it is if you rip it away from them in a game of tug-of-war.

The label can even fail to work with clients who are legitimately dealing with an addiction. Clients can often feel coerced to participate in therapy. They can also feel coerced to take on this label. Many of these people might play roles to satisfy therapists and partners. That may seem harmless, but playing inauthentic roles usually leads to resentment, which can increase the risk of acting out.

Myths, Sexuality Bias, and Other Important Considerations

Myths and bias further muddy the waters when assessing for sex addiction. Unfortunately, many professionals assign the sex addiction label for behaviors that don't warrant it. There are several situations when clients are at risk of being wrongfully called sex addicts. We'll be discussing various situations throughout this book. In my opinion, the most frequent, inappropriate use of this label is with those who view pornography.

As a therapist, you will have your own beliefs about pornography use. You might believe that watching porn is never healthy or appropriate. This doesn't mean that when people use it, it's automatically a sign of an addiction.

Pornography is complicated and difficult to define. It encompasses so many different elements and issues. Porn is also intertwined into several cultural aspects. Some of this I'll be discussing in this book.

I bring the issue of pornography up at this point in this book because I've seen the addiction label being used inappropriately many times. This represents therapist biases. Porn-related problems are often related to communication and boundary issues within a relationship, rather than an addiction to pornography. When you suggest that there is a porn addiction, you have to make sure there is a pattern of out-of-control behavior. You also have to be sure that you're not just promoting your own boundaries. Unfortunately, I've seen therapists call clients porn addicts when there was no pattern of out-of-control behavior.

Over-pathologizing porn use is only one example of how bias can lead to inappropriate labeling. Biases can occur with all of the vulnerable groups discussed in this book. Again, it's not bad to be biased—it's human. It's more important that you're aware of your biases. When you're practicing good awareness, you can better assess the problem and walk with your clients through their journeys.

Our clients come into our offices with a long list of moral, religious, and cultural backgrounds. Their experiences can encourage them to over-pathologize their own issues. Therapists have to hold an even more delicate balance with these clients because they can be easily shamed for their experiences. Sadly, this can lead them to therapists who also have rigid perspectives. More specifically, it can send them to therapists who use shame as a treatment intervention.

Apart from bias, there are several other misunderstandings about addiction that can be confusing to us as professionals, as well as to our clients. The most common myth that I've seen in clients is that they believe that desiring a lot of sex is the same thing as a sex addiction. Other than this, there are other misunderstandings that may come up during therapy. If the timing is right, we can offer gentle education about sexual fantasy and desire, which can help normalize sexuality. Normalization can also help decrease sexual shame. When you hear a client bring up a myth about sexual addiction, assess the level of trust that you've built. Share educational information as it's tolerated, and then use that information to discuss their feelings about the previous misunderstandings.

Shame, Vulnerability, Connection and Addiction

Shame is a very critical element of sexual compulsivity and sexuality in general. We all have the need to connect. Shame is a reflection of that need. It has the potential to make any of us feel unworthy of connection with other people if we let it.

The clients categorized as vulnerable groups in this book are at a higher risk of being shamed for who they are. Many of these clients have a high sensitivity to the biases of others in their lives. Thus, they're often more sensitive to bias and judgment from their therapists as well.

Shame and vulnerability are critical elements to the treatment of sex addiction. Brené Brown's research on shame and vulnerability has brought needed attention to the role of these things in peoples' lives. We continue to learn more and more about how a lack of connection increases the risk for isolation, emotional problems, and addiction issues. We're also learning how shame can contribute to minority stress. Therefore, there is a lot of information about the role of shame and vulnerability in therapy throughout this book.

For now, I want to focus on the general role that shame and vulnerability have on compulsive behaviors. Both of these things can lead to maladaptive coping patterns that increase the risk of addictive behavior. In order to feel a connection, we have to be ready to take chances. We have to be willing to be vulnerable. However, we can often experience shame in our failed attempts at vulnerability as well.

In my experience, shame and vulnerability are critical to the assessment and therapeutic processes. Most of our clients have an authentic need for connection. Every person who is dealing with sexually compulsive behavior struggles with tolerating vulnerability. The only time this isn't true is when you're working with a client who is sociopathic.

The struggle with vulnerability works against our clients' inherent needs to connect. Even when people completely avoid being vulnerable, they still have that need to connect with others. This is how maladaptive coping enters so many of our clients' lives. There's only one pathway to connection, and it's through the scary corridor of vulnerability. In order to feel connected to others, we have to be willing to share information about ourselves. This can be risky. The people we share it with might not accept us. In other words, when we take these chances, we might walk away feeling hurt or rejected.

These are the types of risks that are worth taking. Even though we'll sometimes get hurt, we'll build some connections. We'll learn from it too. That is why I call these *mindful risks*. It's scary and we're taking chances when we do it. However, the risk is worth it because of the potential rewards: connection, feeling seen and heard, etc.

Unfortunately, so many of our clients avoid these risks altogether. They associate vulnerability with certain emotional pain. Rather than walking into these territories, they avoid them. Obviously, this doesn't enhance connection. Instead it increases loneliness, melancholy, and other subtle negative feelings. People have to find ways of coping with these negative feelings.

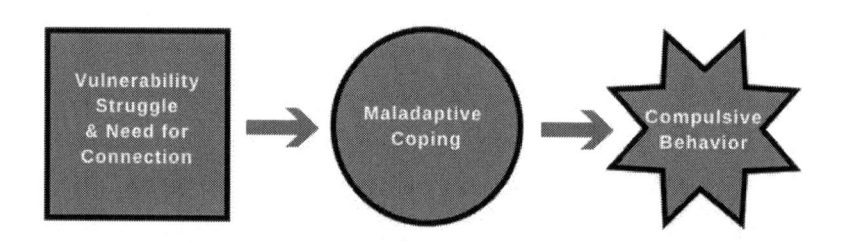

Vulnerability Struggle & Need for Connection → Maladaptive Coping → Compulsive Behavior

Rather than opening up to their support networks, many of our clients cope by utilizing a long list of maladaptive coping mechanisms such as lacking boundaries, numbing, isolating, and avoiding. There are several coping mechanisms that aren't listed here as well. Over time, when specific behaviors are used to deploy these coping mechanisms, compulsive behavior can emerge.

Obviously, these struggles aren't only problems for the vulnerable groups discussed in this book. I believe that shame and vulnerability can be more intense for some of these individuals, because culture has such an impact on shame. A hallmark of addiction is a lack of tolerance of uncomfortable feelings. There are few feelings that are as intense as vulnerability. Therefore, identifying the sources of this feeling can help your clients make changes in their patterns of coping. When feelings are identified, clients can build up an increased tolerance to them. They can also hold a greater appreciation for the positive outcomes of working through failures.

Most of us have learned lessons about vulnerability and connection the hard way. We learn them in childhood and throughout our adulthood. Some are taught to restrict emotions. Others are trained to compartmentalize aspects of their personalities. Then there are those who have made multiple attempts to connect, yet who have walked away from those experiences with serious shame or emotional pain.

Maladaptive coping strategies can become compulsive. They can also co-occur with compulsive sexual behavior. People can struggle to let these behaviors go. Whether a maladaptive coping technique is compulsive or co-exists with other behaviors, it's important for our clients to learn about common reasons for coping in such a way.

Sexual Shame Resilience

Everyone struggles with some level of shame when discussing sex. Sometimes shame appears as that typical, shrinking feeling where we get very small, silent, and even invisible. Other times, shame can be seen in defense mechanisms of attacking others, blaming, lying, and pointing fingers. Whether it's desires and fantasies, or a sexual addiction itself, shame is part of almost everyone's sexual experience. In therapy, we have to help people understand these parts of their stories.

Shame resilience isn't about ridding people of their shame. It's about helping them identify and tolerate it. When people identify shame, it becomes more manageable. They can reach out to their support systems and share their stories. They can also realize that they aren't alone in dealing with situations in their lives

When assessing our clients, we need to monitor for shame resilience. Poor shame resilience can increase the risk of addictions. It can also increase the risk of mood problems, which are also highly correlated with addictive behaviors. I regularly ask clients about their understanding of shame. I also ask people how they've coped with this in the past. When I'm working with sex addiction cases, I specifically monitor for numbing because this can increase the risk of engagement in compulsive behavior.

We live with a lot of sexual paradoxes in our culture. Sex is a type of connective expression. However, we're also taught shameful lessons about sex and eroticism. This leaves a lot of people unclear of what to share and expose. People often feel too vulnerable to share parts of their sexual selves with their partners. This can also make it difficult for our clients to talk about sex in therapy.

When people avoid sharing parts of who they are, it can lead to increased secrecy, isolation, and loneliness. It can even become an emotional source for several of the sexual behaviors that lead to relationship betrayal. These are the situations that we regularly work with in therapy.

Numbing as Maladaptive Coping

People who experience high levels of shame and who have low levels of resiliency are more likely to numb. Therapists need to help clients identify whether or not this numbing becomes pervasive in their lives. All of us numb to some degree. You probably won't have to look too far into your past to find a time when you've used some external source as a numbing agent. Whether it's food, your phone, sweets, or television—we all do this at some point.

For some, numbing behavior goes to another level. For these people, this coping mechanism is over-utilized. It becomes too heavily relied upon as a way of coping with emotions, relationships, and even life. Some can even become so dependent on this that they can't deal with their lives without dipping into their numbing agents.

Five Points to Divide the Lines on Sex Addiction

As you've read, I am encouraging you to balance the benefits of utilizing a label, while also accepting the limitations of it. Labels help with case conceptualization, while also having limited value within the therapeutic setting. Despite my belief of this limited value, I know that many clinical enthusiasts will want more information to help with identifying when clients are genuinely dealing with an addiction. The most obvious times when the label holds value in therapy sessions are when clients identify with it.

Does using the label mean your client is an addict? Not necessarily. However, when clients believe that they're addicts, therapists need to have enough respect to listen to them, so that it's clear how this conclusion was reached. Listening to clients with an open mind helps them develop meaning and build a narrative of personal understanding.

It's important to identify the borders of the sex addiction label when working with vulnerable populations and individuals. As you well know, our case conceptualizations don't always match up with what clients believe about themselves. If there is a discrepancy, this can impact the therapeutic experience. I'll be discussing clients mislabeling themselves, along with how to handle this, throughout this book.

Our clients are often going to believe that their behavior is compulsive. There is a lot of information out there for them to look at. Some of it is good and some of it is poor. Like other situations where clients self-diagnose, some of them will be correct in their diagnosis, while others will not. To help delineate the difference, I've identified five elements that I've observed in every sex addiction case that I've worked with. For many of our clients, information about the behavior itself isn't enough to feel confident that sex addiction is the problem.

These five elements can help you further validate and invalidate a sexual addiction label in your clients. Some of these elements are going to seem obvious. Other points on this list are ones that we have already discussed. I'm again adding them here to help you further divide the lines of addiction in your assessment process.

The five points below can help you separate clients who are coming into therapy for sexual miscommunication, confusion about their relationships, and confusion about their sexuality and gender, from those who are dealing with a genuine addiction. There are times when issues intersect. In these situations, clients may be dealing with an addiction, as well as coping with sociocultural, sociosexual, or gender concerns. This will be discussed at greater length in the following chapters.

Do you have to see all five of these things before validating the existence of a sexual addiction? In my opinion, the answer is "yes." Some of these elements are easier to identify than others. When working with a client, there are certain traits you can see immediately, while others require you to get to know the client before identifying them. Here are those five points:

1. Compulsive sexual behavior.

This might seem like the most obvious element. However, as previously discussed, therapists sometimes allow their biases to affect their diagnosis, thereby leading them to inappropriately use the sex addiction label. When a client is disturbed by their sexual behavior, it requires careful assessment. In the assessment process, you must identify a repetitive, out-of-control behavior pattern to justify the use of the sex addiction label.

It may sound straightforward, but it's not always easy to identify when a behavior is out of control. Identifying how much of a behavior is "too much" is a challenge. These identification issues also exist when identifying problems with other addictions such as substance abuse. When assessing our clients, we have to pay attention to each client's experience and the consequences that are identified.

> **A Note About Partners Diagnosing Clients**
>
> Sometimes clients do come into therapy purely at the request (and even threat) of a partner. The partner may label their behavior as addictive. Clients often label themselves to match their partner's perception of their behavior. Many of the people we work with are in the midst of highly tumultuous emotional situations. They're often dealing with betrayal and severe trauma. Similar to clients who self-diagnose, partners are also often correct about their diagnosis of our clients. However, sometimes this label is given, even though there is no pattern of compulsive behavior. There is a lot for therapists to respectfully juggle in these situations. They have to respect a hurt partner's feelings. Therapists also have to help clients discover self-acceptance and increase their levels of openness.

You're also likely to come across clients who are disturbed by particular behaviors or even fantasies, yet who aren't engaging in a repetitive pattern. To them, the disturbing part of their story may be an internal need for authenticity that is incongruent with their outward relationships and expression. These clients may still call themselves addicts. In these situations, the goal is to offer affirmative support while staying out of a power struggle.

2. Difficulties with establishing connection.

Authentic connection requires interpersonal exposure. This openness requires vulnerability and a tolerance of the feelings that come with it. All of the sex addict clients who I've worked with have struggled with vulnerability. These clients struggle with sharing themselves with the people around them.

Despite this struggle, humans are still built for connection. When people lack a regular sense of connection in their lives, there is an increased risk of emotional, relationship, and behavioral problems. Sexual compulsivity is one of the problems that can develop. Those who struggle to establish and maintain connections have a higher risk of sexual addiction.

Compulsive sexual behavior can stem from a lack of authentic connections. It can also come from regular numbing from an unrecognized need for connection. Either way, I've never met a client who is dealing with a sexual addiction who also feels content with the connections in their lives. These issues can exist within friendships and romantic relationships.

3. Compartmentalization.

Compartmentalization of difficult situations, conflict, and discomfort is another element I've noticed in all of my clients who have dealt with sexual compulsivity. Compartmentalization often includes avoidance and disconnection from stress or life's difficulties. Home-life and work-life can be compartmentalized in different, rigid mental spaces. When difficult emotions are experienced, they can be pushed into compartments as well.

In addictions, these compartments can be utilized to contend with the idea of living a double life. People who are engaging in addictive behaviors often step outside of their values systems. In these situations, compartmentalization is used to box up behaviors such as cheating, lying, and engaging in multiple affairs. These boxes can then be pushed out of that person's mind. People can then avoid dealing with the discomfort of what is inside these boxes. Sometimes this is so powerful that clients may convince themselves that those compartmentalized boxes don't exist at all. This also helps people avoid difficult feelings like shame.

4. Low emotional tolerance to negative emotions.

Tolerating negative emotions is a very difficult task for anyone who is dealing with an addiction. Sex addiction is no different. Mindful coping skills are needed to stay regulated when dealing with negative emotions.

It's also important to learn how to listen to these emotions because they communicate important messages to us. Those who chronically avoid emotions are likely to suffer the consequences of this. Chronic avoidance can lead to further life issues, isolation and relationship problems.

5. Low shame tolerance.

Yes, I know—shame is a negative emotion and I already talked about emotions. However, when it comes to sex addiction, I think shame deserves its own spot on this list. Shame is something that we all experience. We often associate shame with the emotional after-effect of stepping outside of our values. However, it can be a precursor to withholding information as well. Shame can make you doubt yourself and avoid the vulnerability that would have otherwise led to connection.

For those who are dealing with sexuality problems, shame is almost always lingering around. Every culture has some element of shame associated with sexuality, which comes from social norms, misinformation, etc. This emotion can reflect incongruences in the way our clients express their sexuality.

Just as I discussed earlier, people who live with sexual compulsivity can also struggle to tolerate shame. Our clients often come into our offices already facing the toll that shame has taken on their lives. Sometimes they won't even recognize that this is happening.

What Doesn't Matter

Over the years, I've met several therapists who overestimated the influence that they have on their clients' lives. They were educated and trained to believe that they needed to be experts to help people. I'm not trying to shame therapists who are trained in this way because I was one of them as well. Clients came into my therapy office for help with their problems. I simply wanted to help, and I believed that expertise was the key ingredient to offering this. I know I'm not the only therapist who has faced this expectation. Leaders in our field and the media can feed into unrealistic beliefs about our roles as therapists.

We work and train hard throughout our education, internships, and post-graduate training to learn everything we can about mental health, addictions, behavioral concerns, etc. Our backgrounds give us extensive knowledge and experience. This education offers us the skills to utilize different approaches to help our clients. It also helps us conceptualize their cases with our knowledge base.

I'm similar to many of my colleagues. I love to learn. I enjoy gaining insight into new ways of conceptualizing cases. I also love the field that I'm in, so it's exciting for me to grow from trainings; however, conceptualization skills are limited in their value.

I want to share a story with you about how and why my perceptions on expertise have changed. During my educational experience, I had a wonderful mentor who challenged my ideas on the importance of expertise. In one of our consultations, I was processing a complicated case with her. It involved a couple who was struggling to reconnect. I so wanted to help them, but it just wasn't happening. While discussing this case, I went deeper and deeper into the conceptualization, while sharing my thoughts on what was happening in their lives. I just knew that my expertise and training could get this couple to reconnect. Out of nowhere, my mentor stopped me and said, "Michael! Stop... It doesn't matter." I was floored. How could it be that my assessment of this case didn't matter?

I knew that I was spot-on in my conceptualization of the case. In fact, my mentor told me, "Your conceptualization is brilliant... and you know what? It doesn't matter." I understood the struggles that were preventing this couple from reconnecting. Regardless of how much I understood, the truth was that I wanted them to move to a place where they weren't ready to go. While my expertise could help these clients process their situation, it was up to them to turn their relationship into what they wanted it to be.

Our clients have all kinds of people in their lives who know them way better than we do. Many of these people have given them advice and shared their opinions. They have access to different perspectives via the media, etc. There are other dynamics at play that go well beyond our expert advice.

Several of our clients aren't sure why they're coming in to therapy. They know they don't feel well or that they have a crisis to manage. They don't know where to turn, so they come to us for help. Our experience and training can help them. Ultimately, clients will decide on their goals and identify their own needs for therapy.

How is this relevant to sexual addiction? When we rely too heavily on our clinical opinions, we can close doors rather than help our clients open them. Some clients will take on labels. Others will not resonate with them at all. I've worked with clients who have been negatively impacted by therapists who didn't recognize when their advice wasn't needed. Even worse, there have been times when the advice was harmful. In sex addiction therapy, I'm aware that therapists on both sides of the sex addiction argument often try to make their clients see the debate from the therapist's truth.

There are so many problems with this. The first issue is the increased likelihood of the client moving onto another therapist. Some will permanently abandon therapy after a negative experience. Although we're not responsible for our clients' future choices, we have a lot of influence on their perspectives of therapy. Sadly, there are clients who give up on our field when they have a bad experience. When therapists insist on sitting in an expert position in therapy, the probability of these experiences increases.

The second issue involves invalidation. Our clients' experiences have to be respected. It doesn't mean we have to always agree with them. However, when we insist on making them take on a label or a goal that doesn't resonate with them, their process becomes interrupted. For others, their therapeutic process is also affected when we strip them of a label that they're identifying with.

Lastly, when therapists overstep their boundaries, it can throw the therapist into a role where they don't belong. Even when their intentions are good, therapists can wreak havoc and contribute to gaslighting. They can also triangulate the therapeutic relationship to make a point about therapeutic controversies.

Am I saying that you need to avoid conceptualizing your client cases? Of course not. We have to utilize our education and theories to know what to say or do in sessions. We need to know when our clients are in a crisis, or when they need open spaces to walk through their problems. However, we also have to recognize when our expertise is limited.

I encourage you to identify what doesn't matter in your therapeutic processes. You'll likely discover that your knowledge isn't as important as your presence, intent, and acceptance. When it comes to hot topics like sex addiction, it's always tempting to take a side. Like all journeys of personal growth, our clients are going to come into therapy with theories about their situations. We need to be prepared to walk on these journeys with them rather than be bound to our conceptualizations, opinions, and biases. This allows them to identify their own goals and gives them space to change their goals throughout their therapeutic process.

Vulnerable Groups

In sex addiction therapy, some groups are especially vulnerable to being shamed or mistreated for normal expressions of sexuality and gender. Some of these groups can be shamed because of their gender identity or sexual orientation. Others can be shamed or labeled because of their relationship style or desires. I've identified three groups that I believe are the most vulnerable to receiving sex addiction treatment when it's unwarranted. Some of the most significant criticisms of sexual addiction treatment are related to the treatment, and mistreatment, of these particular groups.

Here are the vulnerable groups I'll be talking about throughout this book:

- LGBTQ clients.
- Those who are in non-monogamous relationships.
- People with attraction and desire that can be described as kink, BDSM, and "fetishes."

Even though SOCE practices are more often denounced, LGBTQ individuals are sometimes treated for sexual compulsivity when it's unwarranted. There are various journeys of self-discovery in sexuality and gender expression. There are also several struggles with religious upbringings and social constructs that can occur. Sadly, these struggles continue to bring many people into therapy with the hope of changing this part of who they are.

Individuals with interest in kink or BDSM, as well as those who live with "fetishes," may also come into therapy for sex addiction. Sometimes this behavior may become compulsive. However, the mere existence of such desire and behavior doesn't constitute an addiction. I've worked with people who have been told by therapists that their desire is unhealthy and addictive, when it wasn't compulsive at all. This leads to increased feelings of shame, social isolation, and difficulties with relationships. Being sex positive offers clients a space where they can further understand their desires, develop boundaries, and increase their self-acceptance.

Finally, those who are interested in non-monogamous relationships are often labeled as sex addicts as well. Therapists can hold different biases against open relationship styles. Those who desire polyamorous, swinging and open relationships can be made to feel that their consensual relationship choices are inherently unhealthy. Even worse, they can be told that they're demonstrating "addict behavior" when they're being open about their desires.

Barriers to Being Sex Positive

Sex positivity will be discussed in greater depth later in this book. In identifying a sexual addiction, it's important to name barriers that prevent therapists from practicing sex-positive therapy. Therapists are often unaware of their biases. Many of us work to be congruent with who we want to be, and most of us want to be non-judgmental. However, therapists also regularly over-estimate their ability to work with clients without judgment. Sex positivity isn't about being non-judgmental with no biases to speak of. Being an unbiased human is an unreal construct. Instead, being sex positive is about being aware of your biases. Awareness separates those who practice cultural competency and sex-positive therapy from those who unintentionally harm their clients.

Therapists have to practice developing their sense of self-awareness. This can become a difficult and uncomfortable process. Some studies have even suggested that therapists who are overly confident in their abilities may actually be ineffective and even harmful. You have to look at uncomfortable, personal realities about who you are and what you struggle with in order to best help your clients. It also means that you have to identify your limitations.

A lack of self-awareness can lead to over-diagnosing problems and an overinflated sense of superiority in therapists. Sex-positive therapy is integrative and client-driven. Therapists bring their expertise, but the client determines how this applies to their lives. No therapist has the sole pathway to treat, cure, or identify any problem relating to sexuality. This includes sex addiction. Sexuality involves values systems, culture, and meaning. In cases of sexual compulsivity, we have to value all of these complex human aspects.

Bridging the Divide: Putting Down Weapons and Armor to Help Those in Need

Most people in the field of counseling and psychotherapy have a genuine interest in helping those who are struggling. However, as helpers, we're also human. It's easy for us to lose ourselves in the passion of helping others, especially when discussions surround political and controversial topics. Like everyone else, we have opinions and beliefs. We also have our own stories. These dynamics can lead to tension when controversial topics are involved, and especially when politics and religion are involved.

As you've read, it's impossible to completely separate politics from the topics of sexuality and sexual addiction. We bring our personal biases, our past experiences, and our current perspectives with us everywhere we go. These things come into our therapy sessions too. At the same time, it's important that we avoid pushing our perspectives about sociological issues onto individual clients. Clients may decide that they want to change social structures in a way that is most congruent to them. Therapists are responsible for helping clients identify authenticity and congruency for themselves.

Various political positions and controversies can impact the therapeutic process for the groups discussed in this book. Helping clients identify authenticity and congruency can be difficult. In each chapter, we will look at social barriers to consider for these cases, along with various approaches for contending with these barriers in a way that respects client autonomy and self-determination.

In general, therapists need to remain mindful of sociological interventions when dealing with the following list of issues in therapy. It's not surprising that many of these topics also can influence therapeutic outcomes in cases of sex addiction:

- Religion
- Culture
- Politics
- Childhood and Adolescent Sexuality
- Race/Ethnicity
- Sexual Orientation
- Gender Identity
- Healthy Sexuality
- Relationship Structures
- Non-Traditional Sexual Behavior

Although awareness of social issues is important, therapists must also pay attention to one of their most basic therapeutic rules. Therapists have to ask themselves if the information that they're seeking is something they *need to know* or if it's something they just *want to know*. When information is something therapists want to know, they may be preventing client autonomy. Therapists sometimes engage in small talk to build rapport, but even this is a tool to build and maintain the relationship. Small talk also adds balance to therapy, which can be challenging for clients. Ultimately, therapists need to be aware of the intention behind their questioning and approaches.

In order to be sex positive, therapists must also avoid focusing too heavily on judgmental dichotomies. They need to proceed with caution when they start to classify client behaviors as *right* or *wrong*, and *good* or *bad*. These judgments can cause problems with already established attachment patterns in our clients. They're also sex negative. Judgement that comes from extreme thinking can prevent clients from determining their own therapeutic, life and relationship goals.

Issues such as these can create personal, passionate feelings in all people. Therapists can experience these feelings just like anyone else. It's incredibly important that we remain aware of them. When we're unaware of the impact of our political and religious perspectives, we risk harming our clients. We have to practice a high level of awareness of ourselves and how we view sexuality, sexual orientation, and gender. Many times, therapists feel that they have "no biases" surrounding these things. Similar to issues regarding race, we all have biases. To effectively work with sexuality, it's essential to be familiar with your perceptions, beliefs, and biases.

3

Considerations for Sexual Orientation and Gender

Psychology has a long history of shaming and even abusing lesbian, gay, bisexual, queer, transgender, and non-binary individuals. Several therapists continue to hold shaming perspectives on sexual orientation, gender variance, and gender non-conformity. Some of this shame is a direct response to religious and fundamentalist perspectives. Shame for LGBTQ people also comes from living in a social structure that still reinforces inequality, stereotypes, and myths.

Our society has been making ongoing progress in de-stigmatizing and de-pathologizing variances in gender expression and sexual orientation. LGBTQ people can be more open than ever before. This sense of progress doesn't erase a long history of painful discrimination and abuse, unfortunately. It also doesn't erase the current ongoing issues and challenges that these individuals face in our society. It can still be difficult for LGBTQ people to accept themselves and be open about who they are.

Sex addiction is an especially controversial topic as it relates to gender and sexual orientation. Fundamentalist therapists regularly view gender variance and non-heterosexuality as behavior problems.

They often label LGBTQ people as addicts. This mishandling of the sex addiction label, along with psychology's long, shameful history of treatment of LGBTQ people make it very important to remain mindful when working with these individuals.

I'm going to spend a lot of time talking about bias in this chapter. Therapists have a responsibility to find a balance in their work with their clients. This includes listening to their clients' stories, and also allowing clients to assign their own goals. Bias is something that can influence therapists' work because it shapes our perspectives. It also can influence when and how we intervene with our clients.

The Harmful Effects of Binary Thinking

I believe that our culture is wired for binary thinking. Just look at our political system and sociocultural debates. It's wired within us to want things to be as simple as possible. In general, people also prefer to limit categories so that there are fewer of them to understand.

In our culture, sexual orientation is mostly seen as two opposite categories: straight and gay. When people don't fall into these categories, they're often treated with suspicion and judgment. Those who identify as bisexual, asexual, queer, and fluid are ostracized inside and outside the LGBTQ community. When it comes to sexual orientation, people who are accepting of homosexuality and heterosexuality are often much less accepting of other orientations. This can be isolating for some clients, and can even be discouraging and shameful for others.

Gender is similarly treated in a binary way. In fact, I believe that binary thinking about gender is even more rigid. Physicians and therapists often stand in the way of clients who are transitioning when the client doesn't fit into traditional "male" or "female" categories of identification. Even worse, these clients are sometimes pushed to take on gender pronouns and identities that don't feel authentic to them. I have friends, clients, and colleagues of mine who have been driven into identities that don't fit. I've heard many people share stories of how this has happened to them. This can cause a lot of pain and makes journeys toward self-acceptance even longer and more complicated.

As therapists, we're just as vulnerable to supporting binary schemas and bias. Although I've seen these mistakes made by conservative therapists, I've seen therapists who identify as "sex positive" make mistakes in this arena as well. When our clients don't feel authentic in the binaries that have been established by our society, they're likely to face suspicion. For example, I've seen therapists accuse non-binary people of being confused when they weren't confused at all. In reality, it's often the therapist who is confused. In these situations, therapists are speaking from their own biases when they give this type of feedback.

Bisexual, pansexual, and sexually fluid people can also face several challenges within the LGBTQ community. LGBTQ peers can demonstrate similar binary thinking about gender and orientation. This can be very isolating and shameful for people who face suspicion from a community who is supposed to be supportive.

I'll be discussing LGBTQ biases and assumptions throughout this chapter. In general, the less binary a person identifies, the more challenges they're likely to face. Stereotypes are often hurtful to people and they can also make their journeys more confusing. As therapists, we can offer help to overcome these stereotypes by providing empathy, openness, and a space for personal reflection.

> We can be a validating force in a world full of binary thinking. However, to offer validation, we must be willing to deal with our own assumptions and biases.

The Painful World of Assumptions

Our culture is obsessed with outing LGBTQ people. The phrase, "come out" is reserved primarily for those in the LGBTQ community. For example, people are never outed as straight or cisgender. In our culture, the curiosity about others' sexual orientation often becomes more important than a respect for their privacy. Gender and orientation are used as common materials for gossip columns and celebrity news.

Curiosity about orientation becomes such a powerful force that people enjoy guessing other peoples' orientation. Although doing this may seem harmless, these assumptions are based on stereotypes. People indirectly promote sexual orientation and gender hierarchies by playing these guessing games. In these hierarchies, heterosexuality and cis-genderism sit firmly on top, with homosexuality a step below. Those who are queer, transgender, bisexual, gender-queer, asexual, non-binary, fluid, etc., can be pushed to the bottom. This promotes even more silence, shame, and personal rejection in LGBTQ individuals. Sadly, people are often unaware that they have such an influence on these structures.

Similarly, people also make assumptions about gender. We live in a world of cisgender schemas. These schemas tell us that gender should be easy to identify and label. They also tell us that gender should be assigned by the world around us, rather than by individuals. There are several harmful consequences to these beliefs that can impact people, yet these consequences aren't experienced by cisgender people. Therefore, it can be difficult for them to understand the experiences of non-cisgender individuals.

Gender expression is very individualized. Affirming gender expression should be the aim of all therapists. Affirmation of gender requires us to respect non-linear journeys. When therapists achieve this with their clients, they respect individual journeys of each person, rather than prescribe a journey that matches cultural expectations.

The same is true of sexual orientation. It's also individualized in its expression and journey towards authenticity. Some will come out to others, while others won't. All of these journeys are a personal process. When therapists work with members of this community, it's important for them to work towards being affirmative of their clients. Affirmation involves acceptance of all individual experiences.

Sexual orientation and gender hierarchies are well established in our culture. Unfortunately, if you think you never believe in these schemas, you're likely helping build the foundation that supports them. You have to identify the assumptions that you're most vulnerable to thinking. This awareness will help you stay with your clients through their search for authenticity.

Sex Addiction Therapy with LGBTQ Clients

I know I've already discussed several of the cultural issues surrounding sex addiction and LGBTQ clients, but I need to restate some of them again here. Reiterating these points is important for drawing lines in sex addiction treatment. Historical and societal traumas, along with ongoing cultural changes, biases, and discrimination make sex addiction a controversial topic for LGBTQ clients.

The cultural issues that impact our LGBTQ clients the most are based in fundamentalist, religious perspectives. Religious traditions can lead to fighting against sexual orientation and gender variance. Various religious groups can treat these aspects of people as behavior problems. These groups also show a lack of interest in gaining a better understanding of LGBTQ people, which can lead to further cultural invalidation of these people.

Several of these fundamentalists lead ongoing efforts to change orientation and gender to fit traditional roles. In these efforts, they regularly label variances in gender and sexual orientation (those outside of heterosexuality and cis-genderism) as addictions. These fundamentalists also fail to offer sincere help of any kind. As someone who has worked with many clients who have been in these programs, I can say with confidence that these programs lead to trauma and shame.

SOCE programs continue to exist because of societal and cultural judgment and stigma. Thankfully, these programs are more consistently closing down. They're also becoming illegal in several states. Still, shame continues to lead people to therapists who claim that they can change orientation and gender.

Shame can lead LGBTQ people to our offices as well. I'm always relieved when a struggling LGBTQ client enters my office. It's not the struggle itself that I'm relieved by. I know that we may be in for a long road of sorting out confusion and fear. Rather, I'm relieved because I know that they're in an affirming place. Helping these clients while they're on their path can be tough and even painful, but

I'm also honored to be able to help. Offering this space also prevents them from seeking out help from therapists who can harm them with SOCE.

Respecting Societal Shame and Helping Rather than Hindering

For LGBTQ clients who come into our offices for help with sex addiction, we have another delicate balance to manage. We have a responsibility to help these clients separate out-of-control behavior from authentic needs for self-expression. Although there are times when this is straightforward, there are many other situations that are more complicated.

All of our LGBTQ clients can be at various stages of their journey. Some of these clients are married in same-sex/gender relationships, while others are in mixed-orientation marriages. Some need to process elements of their gender expression. Others will identify themselves as transgender. There are also clients who end up working with us because they're confused about their sexual orientation and gender.

Again, our goal in working with this group is to be affirmative. But what does it mean to be an affirming therapist? To be affirming, we have to encourage authenticity in our clients. We also have to respect the challenges that are ahead of them. A lack of love and belonging, and a fear of losing it, can create significant distress in LGBTQ people. Thus, some of those who seek out therapy want to rid themselves of their need for authentic expression. They might even want us to help them change their orientation or gender to fit the norms of their families, religious organizations, work, and other groups. Therapists can be put into complicated situations. Obviously, we don't want to promote a change in orientation or gender, but some of these clients have extreme anxiety that they believe will only be relieved by a professional who offers SOCE. Therefore, it's important that we offer a space for clients that promotes safety. Otherwise, they're more likely to drop out of affirming therapy and find a licensed professional who offers SOCE.

Good intentions can lead therapists to impede on journeys toward authenticity. We have to allow room for fear, shame, and apprehension to be expressed. I've witnessed therapists allow their passion for the LGBTQ community to impede on individuals' processes. Intense, painful, and complicated situations can be minimized by therapists who intend to comfort their clients. Normalization can help clients, but minimizing struggles in an attempt to comfort usually makes people feel misunderstood.

When working with LGBTQ clients and sex addiction, we also have to be aware of where we refer our clients. A lack of love and belonging is often a source of societal and organizational trauma for our clients. When clients are referred to organizations or groups that fail to treat them with respect, this can enhance these trauma responses.

SOCE groups continue to treat homosexuality and non-cisgenderism as though they're illnesses, bad behavior, and even addictions. SOCE goes against the ethical guidelines of the APA, ACA, and almost every other mental health board. It's a shame-inducing practice that I've seen cause a lot of trauma.

Although Anti-LGBTQ organizations are more regularly prohibited from offering blatant SOCE services to clients they have become more sophisticated in their promotion. Several of these organizations are utilizing key terms that resonate in the fields of psychotherapy and sexuality. I even noticed that one group advertised a mangled version of the definition of "sexual fluidity" as a manipulative tool. Unfortunately, their definition of fluidity was more about leaving room for what they called "heterosexual discovery," than it was about promoting sexual orientation openness and self-acceptance. I've also seen some of these groups offer services claiming that they'll reduce shame. Unfortunately, they believe that they'll reduce shame by eliminating LGBTQ needs for authentic expression. These are dog whistles that are meant to poke at the shame of LGBTQ people while also attempting to sound sex positive on the surface.

These confusing messages can cause a couple of issues for LGBTQ clients. They can create stigma and suspicion around support such as psychotherapy. They also make it complicated for these clients to find safe help when they're trying to separate out-of-control sexual behavior from their needs for authentic self-expression and connection.

Clients often turn to Twelve Step groups for acceptance and support. LGBTQ clients need a place where they can be accepted for who they truly are. As they move through their therapeutic journey, they're more likely to accept their LGBTQ identity (if they hadn't already). When support groups shame their orientation or gender, it can add to their trauma and shame. Again, SA is a Twelve Step group with a definition of sexuality that can be shaming to LGBTQ people. I don't think these clients should be referred to this support group by therapists. At the very least, therapists have a responsibility to warn them about the SA position and the potential harm that it could cause.

That being said, LGBTQ clients often find that support groups are great places for non-judgmental acceptance. With the right social dynamics in place, they can get validation for who they are, while also having a place to process their out-of-control behavior. We can help them find this support in their community by helping them understand when to remain cautious.

We can also help people while they're involved in organizations and groups that don't accept them. I've worked with clients who have come to identify their support groups, churches, etc. as shaming, while they're going through their therapeutic journey. These have been some of the most powerful realizations I've seen in clients. This process can open up doors of true self-acceptance, while also helping clients identify new communities, organizations, and resources where LGBTQ authenticity is valued.

Validating the Experience to Help Almost Any Journey

There are clients who have sex with the same gender, who continue to identify as heterosexual. Some of these clients will identify their behavior as compulsive. This can create a lot of anxiety in therapists who believe in the dangers of SOCE, yet who want to help their clients who lack self-acceptance.

For reasons that I've previously mentioned, SOCE and sex addiction therapy have been conflated by several sex addiction critics. Untangling SOCE from sex addiction therapy is critical for our clients. We need more affirming therapists, not less. When SOCE and sex addiction treatment are conflated, clients may seek out and avoid therapists because of misinformation. This confusion increases the risk that they could end up with a therapist who is harmful or shaming.

The best way to separate sex addiction from SOCE is with unconditional acceptance of our clients. SOCE defines "right" from "wrong." In these situations, the therapist approaches the client's case as if they're the expert in that person's life. From their perception, religious rules are most important. These rules establish the goals of therapy for the client.

Sadly, harming of LGBTQ clients doesn't only come from those who are offering SOCE. I've also witnessed many well-intentioned therapists cause harm to their clients while offering their LGBTQ "friendly" services. Even though these therapists aren't usually bogged down by religious evangelism, they can approach their clients with a similar energy. The therapist is the expert in the client's life. This can lead to inappropriate labeling of that client's sexual orientation, as well as an invalidation of individual experiences.

It's important to differentiate being LGBTQ friendly from affirming. *Friendliness* simply means that the therapist is okay with the client's orientation or gender. The focus is on the therapist's comfort, rather than the client. Whereas *affirming* means that the client feels comfortable with the therapist. Affirmation of the client focuses on the client's identification with their needs and goals. In other words, clients can safely process where they are on their journey and how they identify. They can also openly discuss their emotions and feelings without fear of judgment.

Can you really cause harm, even when you think you're being open-minded? Yes, you absolutely can. All of us have shame. In our culture, shame continues to linger in the lives of LGBTQ people. For some, it's in the periphery. For others, it's blatant and in clear view.

I've seen well-intentioned therapists tell their LGBTQ clients that their orientation or gender isn't a big deal, because it's not something they can change. This is an extremely invalidating approach to helping a client who is being vulnerable. No matter how well-intentioned it is, when you tell clients what their experience should be, you risk shaming them. Instead, we need to ask clients about their experiences and provide validation. Of course, we can ask some challenging questions, but understanding is usually what they need most from you.

The second most common error I've seen by well-intentioned therapists is when they label gender or sexual orientation for their clients. Imagine having shame or fear about your gender or sexual orientation, only to have another person give you a label that doesn't seem to fit. I'm not saying that you shouldn't inquire about your clients' gender or sexual orientation. In fact, I recommend the opposite, which is to avoid assumptions. Asking simple questions can help you see how your clients identify. Respecting this identity can open the door for future realizations, and your clients might be more vulnerable with you and share those realizations as they arise.

Anxiety in Working with LGBTQ Clients

Asking questions can cause a lot of anxiety in therapists when the therapist has a different orientation or identity. This can be extremely anxiety inducing for straight and cisgender therapists. To add to this, there is a fear of asking about clients' orientation or gender because

> it can be perceived as an insult to be questioned about these things. As sexuality professionals, we have a responsibility to change this cultural dynamic as much as we can. We're encouraging it to exist when we avoid these questions.
>
> If you identify as a gender or orientation that is different than your client, it's important to respect the difference. The most basic solution to the fear of stepping into these discussions is to avoid making assumptions. Ask all of your clients about their orientation or gender. This will give you important information about how your clients identify.
>
> When the anxiety is overwhelming, it really means that you need to participate in continuing education and consultation to help you through this. There are several organizations that offer great in-person and distance courses. One of my favorite organizations for courses such as these is the Institute for Sexuality Education and Enlightenment (ISEE). However, there are several other courses out there as well.

When LGBTQ clients struggle with their orientation or gender, shame can make them want to change who they are. How can you affirm someone who wants to change who they are, without accidentally advocating for SOCE? You validate the emotional experience, while practicing authentic acceptance. If the client tells you that they wish they could change their orientation or gender, you can inquire about how that feels. This allows you an opportunity to validate that emotional experience.

All you have to do is hear the stories and feel some of the emotions yourself and it won't be hard to empathize with clients who desire to change the unchangeable. Based on the experiences that people share in therapy, it's understandable that they would want this to be different. They realize how out of control it can feel to have society not accept them, so they're looking to change. Part of their journey will hopefully include a realization that they don't need to change to find love, connection, and acceptance in their lives. We have an important role as therapists to help them navigate through this journey in their own way.

A Note on Straight and Cisgender Clients Who Step Outside of Norms

It's inevitable that you will be working with clients who identify as heterosexual and cisgender, yet who have sex with the same gender, or who step outside of gender norms in some way. Some of these clients will come out later during their therapy journey as transgender, gay, lesbian, or bisexual. They will need your grounded validation while they figure this out for themselves.

There are also other clients who step outside of sexual orientation and gender norms, yet who will continue to identify as heterosexual and cisgender. We have to remain grounded and accept the labels that our clients assign themselves. I've heard several therapists rush to judgment, labeling the orientation of their clients. Doing this can be harmful. Although our culture treats orientation and gender like they should be easy to identify, this isn't always the case. When therapists interfere in this way, or hold these kinds of judgments, they can make their clients' journeys more complicated.

Therapists can help clients make sense of their arousal, expression and orientation. I recommend that therapists inquire about labels, rather than assign them. We can promote self-determination

> by encouraging our clients to share their stories and by helping them establish their goals. Sometimes, we may need to bust myths as they arise. For example, a common myth is that men who wear women's clothing must have gender confusion or must be gay. Another example of a myth is that when men or women have sex or are even attracted to someone of the same gender, they must identify as gay or lesbian. Gender and orientation are complex. Clients and partners sometimes need information about self-expression to bust these myths. Although we can offer education, we also need to let our clients identify their own orientation and gender. With this self-determination, they can also identify the boundaries that make the most sense to them.

Your heart may drop to the floor when you hear some of these stories. Trust me, I know that it can be tempting to want to rescue clients from unaccepting environments and people; however, you have to follow the client through what is important to them. This may include your clients being a part of a family system or religion that is incongruent with who they are. Demonizing their family members and faith will likely lead to premature attrition. On the other hand, if they stay with you, you can help them get through an entire self-acceptance transformation. At the very least, you can plant some seeds of thought for the future challenges that are ahead.

> ### A Different Perspective on Fundamentalism
>
> I advocate for a grounded approach when working with religious fundamentalism. Just like anyone else who is sex positive, I'm deeply saddened by how fundamentalism can hurt our clients. I feel

the need to advocate for those who are hurt by their religions, especially LGBTQ people.

Every time I work with a client who has a history of religious abuse and trauma, I have to remind myself to slow down and stay grounded. Working with fundamentalist clients is a tremendous opportunity to help them look into a mirror with a kind of support that they've never had before. If pushed to look into that mirror before they're ready, I know they're likely to fall out of therapy. When these clients leave an affirming place early, they're at an increased risk of falling into the hands of professionals who won't practice such levels of acceptance.

This type of work requires a great deal of mindfulness. I recommend therapists participate in consultation for these cases, even when you're not in supervision. I still check in with my team on fundamentalist cases to share where I'm struggling and reflect on why this is happening. This also reminds me of how much I can help these clients when they stay in therapy.

Over the years, I've worked with several fundamentalist clients who have moved towards acceptance. I know how important mindful support is to fundamentalist clients because I've had clients validate this. One compliment that I will never forget came from a long-term, transgender client. He told me, "You never told me who I was. You always let me figure it out on my own. I used to get so frustrated with you, but I'm so grateful for it now." In this client's most profound struggle, if I would've told him that he was transgender, he would've disappeared. Even though it was frustrating for him, he was able to move towards self-discovery at his own pace.

Separating Shame from Guilt

Religious fundamentalism can lead to rigidity in beliefs. This is especially true for LGBTQ clients who come from these backgrounds. Therapy has the potential to help clients work towards self-acceptance. It can also open up incongruencies that can be very difficult to face. Therapy also provides a place where clients can have their bravery validated and their shame can be better understood.

Fundamentalists often believe that shame maintains good behavior. I've had several clients who were affiliated with religious institutions that believe that shame is the only way to salvation and happiness. Therefore, these clients can be resistant to shame resilience work. Separating shame and guilt can become even more complicated when shaming belief systems are valued in our clients' family systems.

Shame can lead to increased compartmentalization and increased mood problems. Obviously, it can increase the risk of sexual compulsivity as well. It's a topic that therapists must gently probe with their clients, but it's essential to discuss shame nonetheless.

Over the years, I've discovered that gentle, respectful questioning is the best approach for shame-filled topics. In general, people avoid talking about shame. When clients start to share their stories, they can better identify what is out of control and who they are. They also can build tolerance to discussing shame in their lives. However, it can take time for them to tolerate these conversations.

I also believe it's important to discuss guilt with our clients. This helps them separate guilt and shame. In most cases, I've found that clients are more open to hearing about the harmful impact of shame when this separation is pointed out. This encourages clients to identify their personal values. For example, I've worked with several clients who come out while in heterosexual marriages. Shame leads them to explore their sexuality in secrecy. This can be a heartbreaking situation for so many of these clients and their partners. They really do love their partners and they don't want to cheat on them. They also value holding to their relationship contracts of monogamy. When shame is reframed to guilt, clients can work to understand their incongruencies and begin opening up.

Considerations for Partner Trauma

Some married lesbian, gay, and bisexual clients who are married eventually come out to their partners. Others come out after they have been discovered to have been caught cheating. This creates a very complicated situation with many layers.

When partners discover cheating in these types of situations, they're face-to-face with several issues. First, a person who they've trusted has been discovered cheating. Second, the person hasn't been authentic with them about their orientation. It's understandable why lesbian, gay, and bisexual clients might keep these secrets and lie. Regardless, secrecy and lying also can create a traumatic experience for partners.

When someone discovers cheating or an affair that also leads to questions about orientation, partners can experience a deep level of shame. Some even feel that they're somehow to blame for not only the cheating, but also the other person's orientation. The outcomes from this can lead partners to cope in all kinds of ways. In these situations, the clients we see in therapy will likely be experiencing anger, avoidance, and denial. These are common coping mechanisms.

Some partners battle their own shame by shaming the other person. Others get frozen in the situation. Rather than identify their own needs and boundaries, they put the whole situation out of sight and mind as much as possible.

I believe that boundary and trauma work is crucial with these partners. They have to identify what they want and what is okay with them in the relationship. It's also common for them to require help decompartmentalizing the situation, so that it becomes progressively more tolerable. With a lot of time and help, I've found that these partners are often willing to be supportive of the other person, but this shouldn't be required of them. They have to decide for themselves whether they can sit in that person's support section. Obviously, I recommend that the other person also have their own therapist to navigate through the situation towards self-acceptance as well.

This isn't to say that this makes their journeys easy. Even when the situations are painful, I offer a lot of validation for the bravery it takes to open up. In some situations, clients will be ready to make life-changing, personal changes when they learn about themselves in therapy. Other times, the changes aren't as significant and groundbreaking. In fact, they may go through a journey that is mixed with progress, fear, shame, and joy. No matter where clients end up on their journey, I believe that separating shame and guilt is a critical part of their process.

Confrontation and Boundaries

There are moments when gentle confrontation and boundaries are needed in therapy. Some clients will ask to have their orientation or gender defined for them. Others might ask to be told what to do with their church, family, and work. They might also want a therapist who will tell them that their orientation or gender identity is bad.

To find a balance, I remind myself that these requests come from a place of societal and historical trauma. Empathizing with that trauma helps me stay gentle and understanding, while setting a boundary in session. To do this, I inform clients why I can't tell them what to do with their lives. I also practice empathy with how difficult these situations can be. This practice of boundary is usually a safe way of drawing lines when needed without alienating and isolating a client who is struggling.

Therapist Roles with Sexual Compulsivity in LGBTQ Clients

As you can see, there are various concerns that prompt LGBTQ clients to seek therapy. Some of these clients' problems can be wrongfully labeled as sexually addictive behaviors. Sometimes these clients may be engaging in behavior that is out of control or compulsive. Other times, they might be expressing who they are in the secrecy and silence of shame. Then there are situations where both of these things are true: there is compulsive behavior and a need for authentic self-expression of an LGBTQ identity.

Therapists have a delicate role when it comes to helping clients process all of these circumstances. We have to offer a safe place for our clients to find authenticity and reduce shame. This can be challenging for us when they're also engaging in behavior patterns that are out of control or compulsive. This balancing act takes time and patience, as well as self-awareness as the client's therapist.

Some gay, lesbian, and bisexual clients enter into heterosexual marriages without fully realizing their orientation until they're well into the marriage. Sometimes, these clients will end up cheating. It's important to avoid labeling this cheating as an addiction, unless it's undeniably compulsive in nature.

These clients are also at risk of misinterpreting their issues as an addiction. In these situations, I recommend that you help clients examine their beliefs about why specific behaviors and patterns are addictive. When the only thing that feels out-of-control is an expressive behavior, you may want to further explore this with the client. This can encourage clients to identify their needs and desires, and reframe their own mislabeling.

The process of identifying compulsive sexual behavior can be frustrating when clients are engaging in a compulsive pattern, yet don't see it as a problem. It's a complex process to identify what is out of control. It's challenging to put plans in place to manage any behavior when it's not recognized as a problem.

Building a plan around sexually compulsive behavior, while also helping LGBTQ clients find self-acceptance is a process that can take a long time. Clients with an evangelical history may have the most trouble separating out-of-control behavior from authenticity, but with support and patience, these clients can get to a place where they accept who they are. They're more likely to share it with others as well and find important support systems.

In my experience, clients will likely benefit from processing their feelings and personal understanding before pursuing relationships outside of their marriage. They won't all listen to this advice, however. It's critically important that they aren't shamed for their relationship choices during this time. You can offer recommendations, while also empathizing with your clients' experiences. It's a tough balance for therapists, but it's absolutely necessary when working with clients who have yet to come out.

A Note on Partners and the Family

I believe it's important to try and get the family of LGBTQ clients involved in therapy. You might be the one to provide family therapy to your clients, or you might refer them to a family therapist. This can help the family share their perspectives without shaming the LGBTQ person during the process.

Self-acceptance can be a complicated process for LGBTQ people. This can lead to a variety of experiences for partners. They often have to process their sense of betrayal, fear, and even trauma. At the same time, partners and family members often feel a need to be supportive. Although there are some partners who believe that being LGBTQ is a behavior problem, this isn't true of most. In fact, a lot of partners even feel validated when they finally know the truth.

Knowing that a partner identifies as LGBTQ doesn't make it a less complicated journey, however. Thus, family therapy is the best place for these things to be discussed. The family system will shift with new identities and expression. People have to process and share what they want and how they intend to move forward. They also have to learn how to communicate in the family system without shaming each other.

After authenticity is firmly established, the lines between compulsive behavior and personal identity have to be further separated. This division helps clients identify when their behavior may be compulsive. It can also help to further prevent shame from ruling this person's life. In other words, the whole situation can feel very muddy in the beginning. We can help clients see things clearer over time.

Some clients who have compulsive behavior before coming out will see it diminish or even stop altogether after coming out. Other clients will have compulsive behavior patterns that continue even after they come out. Although this can be very puzzling to our clients, it makes a lot of sense. Again, compulsive behavior is often rooted in maladaptive coping patterns. Maladaptive coping can be rooted in shame and patterns of secrecy. Coming out can help, but it doesn't necessarily erradicate shame from any client's life.

Concerns for Gay and Lesbian Clients and Sexual Compulsivity

Gay men are at a particular risk of being wrongfully labeled as sex addicts. Cultural awareness is a must when evaluating gay and lesbian clients to avoid inappropriately using labels. Again, cultural and societal stigma encourages secrecy and silence. Behaviors can be based in shame without being compulsive at all. For example, a person may engage in behaviors such as lying, having an affair, watching porn in secrecy, etc., without these behaviors representing an addiction.

When a gay, or lesbian client is seeking out your help for sexual compulsivity, you need to be aware of behaviors that are based in cultural shame. For example, the only option for sexual exploration for gay men has sometimes been sex in a public place. Pornography or chatting might be the only way for other people to explore sexuality as well. In some situations, the Internet is the only way for these people to receive sexual education about gay and lesbian sex. In other words, therapists can't draw broad strokes with an addiction paintbrush when dealing with any group, but especially when working with these groups.

A Note About Porn and Gay Men

Gay men, in general, tend to have different perspectives about pornography use than their straight peers. In the heterosexual community, perspectives on pornography are more generally negative. This isn't to say that heterosexual clients will not ever be open to pornography, but it has been my experience that gay men are generally more open about porn in their relationships and tend to feel less negatively about it.

Therapists have to be aware of their perspectives on pornography use and be careful not to shame gay clients who openly use it. Some gay men identify pornography as problematic in their relationships. In these situations, they might feel that it has taken away from their connection. Others consider it to be an authentic element of their sexual expression. Therapy offers a way for clients to make decisions about their boundaries.

Clients who compulsively use pornography tend to have a history of poor sexual education. Gay men are at a higher risk of receiving poor sex education because gay sex and relationships are rarely discussed in these programs. Most sex education programs don't apply to them very well. For many gay men, pornography is a place where they can privately learn about sex without being shamed for their desires.

Pornography has obvious limitations in its efficacy as an educational tool. Clients who have utilized porn as a primary educational tool are at an increased risk of buying into sexual myths. Therapists need to evaluate these clients' past sex education. Doing so opens up a doorway that can build an understanding of the origins of the compulsive behavior and tackle myths as well. This will make therapy a safer place to discuss clients' sexual histories, desires, and the interpersonal impact of their journeys in a safe, affirming way.

Sexual compulsivity is a problem for some gay and lesbian clients. Some of these clients continue certain patterns of behavior, despite ongoing consequences. In these situations, the patterns may become compulsive and pervasive. This can include compulsive sexual behavior and secrets, sexual and relationship avoidance, and even compulsive porn viewing that negatively impacts the clients' relationships. Some gay and lesbian clients have a decrease in problematic behaviors after they come out, but this isn't true for all. Others continue to struggle with ongoing compulsive behavior well after they have come out.

Emotional self-acceptance and self-esteem are important aspects of the therapeutic process for several gay and lesbian clients. Internal dislike, shame, and even hatred are common in these communities. Gay men are at risk of falling into gender role myths of masculinity.

Both gay men and lesbian women are at a higher risk of anxiety and depression that are rooted in a lack of self-acceptance.

Integrative Models for LGBTQ Clients

I have a particular fondness for Gina Ogden's 4-Dimensional Model of sex therapy. It can be beneficial for helping LGBTQ clients explore their personal and sexual stories. In this model, clients share mental, physical, emotional, and spiritual aspects of their sexuality. I've also found it to be a useful tool for working with self-acceptance as well.

This model offers an integrative and fun way for clients to share different aspects of their story. They can also gain some personal insight into meaning, mental messages, and even traumas. Finally, clients who feel stuck or frozen can benefit from literally standing up and walking around while exploring their stories. For more information about the 4-Dimensional Model, please refer to Ogden's book, *Expanding Sex Therapy*.

Trauma therapy can be another critical element of the therapeutic process for LGBTQ clients. Attachment wounds from neglect, bullying, and other types of abuse are common in this community. Some of these things happen because our culture prevents most parents from identifying and addressing LGBTQ developmental needs. There are also some societal and historical traumas that this group can face. Therapists have access to several ways of addressing trauma in therapy, but EMDR and Somatic Experiencing are two approaches that I've found to be most useful.

Considerations for Bisexual Clients

In my experience, bisexual clients may be even more at risk of being shamed by peers, family, friends, and even therapists. Our societal tendency to be binary can make it difficult for people to understand bisexuality. Therapists are no exception to this. Binary thinking can make self-acceptance quite complicated for these individuals.

Bisexual men and women may bury their bisexuality for the acceptance of others. Some spend most of their lives believing that they're straight because they've been only in straight relationships. Therefore, it can be complicated for bisexual people to find validation in their lives. It can also be difficult for them to find understanding and open-minded people for support.

Suspicion and assumptions toward bisexual people are common. Stereotypes and judgments exist even within the LGBTQ community. People often believe that bisexual individuals are really just gay or lesbian people who are in denial. Other people treat bisexuality with suspicion and distrust. Similar assumptions can come from their straight counterparts as well. Sadly, I've also heard these assumptions come from therapists.

People who aren't bisexual also oversexualize this community, while oversimplifying their needs. These individuals are often assumed to be desiring non-monogamy. Relationship styles and sexual desire are as varied among bisexual individuals as they are for anyone else. These assumptions do nothing more than demonstrate judgment.

Affirming therapy helps these clients understand their sexuality and sexual orientation, and how these things relate to their relationships, authenticity, and desires. Our cultural assumptions, schemas, and judgments can lead to feelings of isolation for bisexual clients. Therapists have to practice holding space for these clients, so that these clients can identify what authenticity looks like in their own lives.

Navigating Heteronormativity and Cisgender Bias

Heteronormativity is the normalization of heterosexual trends. To be more specific, it's the normalization of heterosexual dynamics in relationships and sex. A lot of people assume that the roles of masculinity and femininity need to be filled for a relationship to work. Culturally, most people assume that heterosexual norms must exist in same-sex relationships as well. Sexual positions, romance, courtship, and porn usage are all topics where assumptions can take over.

Cisgender bias is the assumption that people naturally have a gender identity that matches their birth sex. This can lead to several assumptions about gender, including binary thinking about gender expression. In cisgender bias, people can be put into categories of "male" and "female," even when it doesn't feel authentic. People may also be assigned a gender category that is inauthentic to them.

These biases aren't something that most people easily see. Most of our relationships are role-modeled from straight relationships. Adults in our culture assume that children will develop into straight adults. Gay, lesbian, and bisexual children are forced to deal with these assumptions throughout their development. For example, adolescents are often asked questions about dating, but the assumption is almost always that they're heterosexual. Few, if any, are asked about romantic interests of the same gender.

Gender variance can also lead to several cisgender assumptions. People stereotype others to match heterosexual constructs. Many are assigned a heterosexual orientation that is assumed to fit their gender identity. All of this can make the journey towards authenticity painful and confusing. Therapists can help this process by remaining aware of their biases, although, they can also hinder this process when they make assumptions.

Our culture and society treat heterosexual and cisgender identities as standard and normal. Orientations and genders that are outside of this are considered different, less common, and even abnormal. Even those who are accepting of LGBTQ people can hold remnants of this hierarchical belief structure. Thus, even when people are supportive, there is still a cultural undertone that remains.

Cultural undertones aren't easily identified. Despite this, they're still powerful. When we treat certain groups as normal, people base their personal assumptions on these schemas. In other words, when you're an LGBTQ person, it can be difficult to see yourself in a heterosexual, cisgender world.

These undertones, along with the blatant discrimination in our politics, churches, etc., can lead our clients to assume they're heterosexual and cisgender, even when they aren't. In these situations, clients may believe that they're "acting out" an addiction, when they're really just expressing a part of who they are.

Men Who Have Sex with Men (MSM)

MSM is a term used to describe men who have sex with other men, yet who also identify as heterosexual. I've seen these men treated with extreme suspicion by laypeople, but by therapists as well. In my experience, this type of bias is primarily reserved for men. We live in a world of cultural assumptions about men's sexuality. When men have any interest in sex with other men, they're usually assumed to be gay.

There are men who begin their coming out process in denial (not being out to themselves). There are also others who currently identify as bisexual, yet later come to identify as gay. However, there are a lot of heterosexual-identified men who have had sex with other men.

Therapists have to remain mindful to avoid assuming that these men are closeted and personally unaware of their orientation. Making these types of assumptions can be invalidating and painful. Instead, they need to be validated in their identification, so that they can sort out their orientation and sexuality in a way that feels authentic to them.

I've worked with clients who've had very shaming therapeutic experiences. Some therapists have even attempted to assign these clients with an orientation that doesn't fit. Inquiring and assuming are very different things and assuming can cause harm. It's always important for therapists to know the difference.

If you find yourself distrusting of a man's insight into his orientation, your distrust is a form of gender bias. It could even be based in sexism and homophobia. For example, we're much less likely to doubt women when they have sex with other women, yet still identify as heterosexual. I would argue that this is based in our culturally-rigid attitudes about gender, sexuality, and the roles of

> cisgender men. Sex positivity is about listening to our clients and allowing them to figure out their stories, sexuality, and lives.

To manage the rigidity of gender and sexual orientation assumptions, we have to practice slowing down and owning our biases. Our job is to hold space without telling clients who they are and what authenticity should be to them. Clients will come to their own conclusions and identify the labels, or lack thereof, that best suit them.

Mixed-Orientation Marriages

Before discussing dynamics of mixed-orientation marriages, it's crucial to define what it is. A mixed-orientation marriage is one that includes a person who is gay, lesbian, or bisexual and another who is heterosexual. Some of these relationships maintain a sexual component, while many others do not. It's important to note that when therapists recognize and respect these marriages, it's different from SOCE. In these relationships, couples are aware of the differences in orientation and accept them. They choose to remain together while accepting this, rather than promoting sexual orientation change.

Several clients come into therapy with fears of coming out and/or problems with self-acceptance. However, it shouldn't be assumed that people in mixed-orientation relationships have this fear, nor should it be assumed that they're struggling with a lack of self-acceptance. A majority of our gay, bisexual, and lesbian clients will begin to realize that their marriages won't be able to meet their relational and sexual needs, although this isn't true for everyone.

Others choose to stay in their marriages with their heterosexual partners. There are others who decide to stay married for the time being, only to realize down the road that their relationship isn't workable.

Mixed-orientation marriages can come with a lot of judgment. In fact, I've seen some of the most self-proclaimed, sex-positive therapists hold a lot of judgment toward those who are in these relationships. These critical perspectives may feel like they're coming from a place of good intentions. Most therapists wholeheartedly want their clients to find a place of self-acceptance and shared love. It may seem like clients won't find this if they remain in their mixed-orientation marriage. Thus, our visions of an ideal life for our clients can influence the type of guidance we offer them.

There are mixed-orientation relationships that won't work. Over time, many of these couples realize that their relationship needs include sex and romance that isn't possible in the current situation. These decisions can take a lot of time and personal reflection. Social pressures, as well as personal values, need to be processed by everyone in the relationship. Therapists have to be cautious not to shame clients during the process. Values systems don't change overnight. Neither does incongruency. When we push clients too harshly, they're likely to feel judged.

Some mixed-orientation marriages transition into more open-relationship styles. These relationships can include sexually open marriages, as well as more polyamorous relationships. We'll discuss these styles in more depth in a later chapter. We also need to offer a safe space for clients to discuss these options. For example, a mixed-orientation couple may appreciate their reliability, respect, and love. At the same time, they might want open possibilities for sex or other types of experiences with other people outside their marriage.

Mixed-orientation marriages can be very challenging. Therapy can open up lines of communication that help process needs and goals. In fact, I've had clients who've come to realize that their mixed-orientation marriages won't work while they were in couples' therapy. This realization often leads to a smoother transition to life after separation or divorce.

Overcoming Your Biases

All therapists have biases. Conservative therapists may be at risk of treating sexual orientation or gender expression as a disorder. Progressive therapists are at risk of assuming that their comfort is enough to help their LGBTQ clients during therapy.

Affirming therapy for LGBTQ clients requires therapists to have knowledge of their own biases. Looking at yourself is a messy and uncomfortable process. It requires you to walk through the shame of owning biases. The good news is that when you recognize them, you can manage them. However, it's hard to see into your own blind spots. This is why I created the following list of common biases, along with broader considerations to help you tackle each bias along your journey.

Common LGBTQ biases:
- **Sexual position preferences align with traditional masculine and feminine characteristics.** Some people assume that if a gay man is more feminine, then he naturally enjoys being more

sexually submissive or being penetrated. These assumptions can be shaming and flat-out wrong.

- **All LGBTQ people want to get married.** A lot of gay men don't want to be married. Some also don't necessarily want to remain in monogamous relationships. Unfortunately, clients can be pushed into traditional relationship styles by their therapists.
- **Transgender people are also gay or lesbian.** Gender and sexual orientation aren't the same. Gender reflects expression and congruence with an identification, whereas orientation reflects desire, attraction, and romance.
- **Bisexuality doesn't exist.** Unfortunately, people often assume that bisexuality is a myth. People can absolutely be attracted to both men and women. In fact, they can be attracted to many genders.
- **All gay men have penetrative sex.** Sometimes we talk about sexual penetration like this is the only way to connect sexually. There are various ways for people to sexually connect. This is true of gay men as well.
- **Bisexual people are just in denial about their sexual orientation.** Cultural, binary thinking leads people from within and from outside of the LGBTQ community into assuming that bisexual individuals are unaccepting of a gay or lesbian orientation. Although there are some gay and lesbian people who first come out as bisexual, there are also many people who are bisexual and never identify as gay or lesbian.
- **All transgender people want surgery.** People can express their gender in various ways. Be cautious about creating this journey

for your clients. Let your clients identify the best ways to express their gender.

- **Gender transitioning is going from "being a man" to "being a woman."** Authentic gender transitions don't begin with hormones or surgery. It's not an overnight process that reflects only two genders. Clients determine when and how they identify with their gender. Also, this journey isn't a binary process. There are many forms of gender expression and endless genders as well.

This is by no means a complete list of biases relating to sexual orientation and gender. It can be difficult to know if your belief systems are biased or not. Consultation is the answer to this. Good consultation can help you remain grounded to biases and also help you identify ways of addressing these in therapy when they arise.

Helping a Client Who Wants SOCE

LGBTQ clients have the potential to come into therapy with the hope of changing their sexual orientation or gender identity. When we help these clients, we have a delicate balance to navigate. As you have read, my hope is that these clients remain in therapy with an affirming therapist. Obviously, it's unethical to offer SOCE. At the same time, we can still help these clients while they're on their journey. It's important to tell clients how you think you can help, even though you can't provide SOCE. This reminds clients that our goal isn't to force an identity onto them, and it also reminds them that they have a safe place in our therapy offices.

Here are ways in which affirming therapy can help clients who are seeking out SOCE:

- They can learn that they're still in charge of their lives.
- They can be heard and seen.
- They can find hope.
- They can realize their self-worth.
- They can align with honesty.
- They don't have to live in constant fear.
- They can make their own decisions about their places in their families.

Gentle curiosity is my favorite approach to helping clients who want SOCE. In this approach, I focus on inquiring about the different struggles and incongruencies that the client brings up in each session. Gentle curiosity is exactly as it sounds. It is therapists asking curious questions to encourage clients to expand on the beliefs and backstory of their current situations. Sometimes direct confrontation isn't well tolerated by clients who are seeking SOCE. The gentle curiosity approach encourages clients to connect meaning to their religion, shame, morality, sexual orientation, and gender at a pace that they can tolerate. This approach shows them that their therapist isn't judging their answers. It's also accepting of clients who haven't developed solid answers. Last but not least, being curious also gives therapists an opportunity to validate their clients' experiences.

Examples of Gentle Curiosity

The following are examples of gentle curiosity that I have used to help my clients explore their feelings when they desire SOCE:

- What makes you believe that you need therapy to change your sexual orientation or gender identity?
- Where did you learn about sexual orientation or gender expression?
- What emotional words would you use to describe how you're feeling about your sexual orientation or gender?
- What do you think causes differences in attraction?
- What messages were you taught about sexual orientation and gender?

These questions are a basic way of helping LGBTQ clients deepen their personal awareness and self-acceptance. Therapists have to use their therapeutic judgment to identify the best times to ask these questions. There are going to be times when clients can't answer direct questions. Other times, they may legitimately not know the answers. It's important to provide space and give clients the time they need to develop more solid answers. This can take a long time. Gentle curiosity provides this time.

When clients are able to express shame, hurt, anger, grief, and fear, they can receive empathy from their therapists. Empathy is a critical aspect of everyone's process towards self-acceptance, authenticity, and shame resilience. When we provide a space for empathy, it encourages clients to explore their lives and emotions in a progressively open way.

As shame resilience increases, our clients become better equipped to tolerate more education about sexual orientation and gender. I've had clients who struggle with a lack of tolerance for these discussions because of the shame that they feel. I've found that these clients are best able to tolerate these discussions after they've enhanced their trust in therapy, increased social resources, and learned to manage their shame.

When clients progress to accepting their sexual orientation or gender as it is, they can tolerate tougher questions. It's important to remember that some of your clients won't get there while working with you, but you have an opportunity to plant some seeds that can help them on their journey, even if their journey continues with other affirming therapists.

Therapists have to maintain a steady balance to determine when to gently push reluctant clients, while respecting the space and time that clients need. This is why self-awareness is so critical for therapists. Without such awareness, you might become impatient with your client and push too quickly. When this happens, you have to own that you've moved too fast. Demonstrating such vulnerability can build further trust in their journey towards self-acceptance.

Extremes Exercise

Another exercise that I've found useful for clients who are searching for self-acceptance is the Extremes Exercise. I like this because this is an exercise where you stand up and move around the room in therapy. Many of our clients are frozen. They're literally stuck. The fear that comes from strict social constructs can be what is making them feel stuck. Sometimes, sitting in a chair and talking to another person is just not enough to promote moving out of a freeze. This exercise can help them expand on these constructs.

Logic and intense, negative emotions rarely work that well together. LGBTQ clients are often dealing with intense emotions.

We've already talked about shame, which may be the most intense emotion of all. However, there are several other negative emotions that are common as well. When people react to them, it can be difficult for them to make life decisions.

The goal of the exercise is to encourage clients to step away from extremes, while sharing the emotional elements of their story. Clients will often find relief in the middle ground, but it's still scary for them to step away from the extremes. Social pressures promote people to live in constructs and make assumptions about those constructs. People decide how they align with their own identities. However, people also tend to use constructs when they're living outside of authenticity to understand where they are heading. They're trying to make sense of everything. Unfortunately, those constructs often push people to freeze out of fear.

The Extremes Exercise gets clients to literally step out of these frozen spaces. When they take one or two steps away from assumptions, they can share their feelings of fear, powerlessness, hopelessness, etc. They can also get validation from you. At the same time, they're likely going to see and feel what a step towards authenticity is like. I've had several clients who were surprised about how different they feel when they start moving around the room, processing various assumptions about extreme identities, and taking steps away from the extremes.

The middle ground can represent the amount of time it takes this person to find authenticity. It can also help clients see how broad authenticity can be. What represents the middle will be different for each client, which is the beauty of this exercise. They're the ones sharing, experiencing and defining, while you're there to hold space.

Here is an example of how I do the Extremes Exercise. On one end of the room I have clients list constructs, assumptions, and beliefs about being "out" or "open" as a gay, lesbian, bisexual, transgender, queer, or non-binary person. They list their concepts, emotions, and even stereotypes on that end of the room. I encourage people to list rational and irrational elements. In other words, I don't want clients to restrict themselves by being rational.

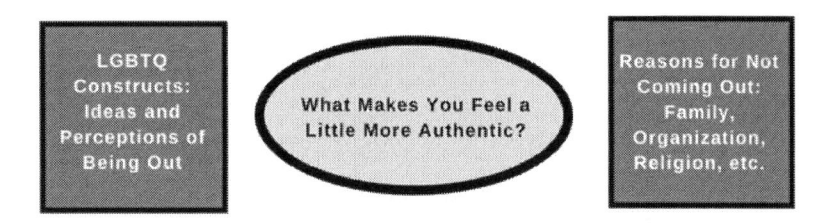

LGBTQ Constructs: Ideas and Perceptions of Being Out	What Makes You Feel a Little More Authentic?	Reasons for Not Coming Out: Family, Organization, Religion, etc.

On the other end of the room, I have clients list aspects that they see as barriers to coming out. In other words, these are the things that make them feel like they shouldn't come out. This can include church, family, and friends. It could also include work and many other organizations. Whatever they choose to list, we talk about the emotions and feelings that are associated with this.

I begin the exercise by having the client stand on one end of the room. Then they discuss the feelings and narratives that represent that side. Keep in mind, this can take an entire session (or more) to process. Some of our clients have experienced a lot of societal trauma, which can open up some serious emotional experiences in this first step.

Then I have clients do the same on the other side. Similarly, they name feelings and narratives that represent that side. They discuss fears, and things that they believe will be different if they aligned with this construct.

After there is a good personal understanding of the extremes, I introduce the center. I don't actually write down "What makes you feel a little more authentic?" in the center. Instead, I start by pointing out the space between the extremes. My favorite question is "I wonder what half a step towards the middle would be like?" I also ask what feelings and emotions they notice when they start to identify the middle ground. This can help clients see more tolerable steps and changes, while still respecting the anxiety that they have.

This exercise provides an opportunity for therapists to point out incongruencies and misperceptions. For example, there may be assumptions that family members are going to be unaccepting. The fear is understandable, but it could be based in a lack of evidence as well. Thus, you can inquire about other more positive possibilities when the opportunity presents itself. Clients often end up uncovering these possibilities for themselves when they step into the center area. Though, sometimes the freeze that they're experiencing can be extremely powerful. Offering other possibilities can sometimes get clients moving a little bit more.

I love the Extremes Exercise when working with clients who are stuck. I have seen it reduce clients' shame, increase their comfort, and identify areas of negotiation in systems that would otherwise be too rigid. I hope it can do the same for you.

Special Considerations for Transgender and Gender Non-Binary Individuals

I have a particular place in my heart for clients who aren't cisgender. As a person who highly values social justice, I find it important to advocate for the most vulnerable. It has been my experience that gender care clients often have to contend with some of the most significant challenges in our society. Members of this group can deal with even more intense feelings of isolation and shame. They also regularly deal with discrimination and transphobia within the LGBTQ community itself.

People often choose therapy as a place to address gender confusion. Those who come to therapy for gender care tend to be misunderstood amongst therapists. Confusion about the difference between gender expression and sexual orientation is quite common. There is also a lot of confusion over sexual, "fetishistic" behaviors and gender variance.

Issues with sex and gender are perpetually intertwined within our political landscape. As therapists, our personal and political opinions can create intense feelings that can impede the therapeutic process. As our political system becomes more extreme, our clients are more likely to be forced to deal with the emotional fallout. I've seen radical politics manifest into intense fear, anxiety, internalized hate, and depression in LGBTQ clients, and especially in my transgender and non-binary clients.

While there are several issues that overtly impact our ideas on gender and human rights, there are just as many covert issues that we have to understand as well. Unfortunately, there is no way to make a complete list of covert beliefs because there are just too many. This is why it's important to continue to gain education and consultation, and continue to ask yourself tough questions to identify beliefs that may cause problems in session. Understanding your perspectives on issues of women's health, gender inequality, sexual assault and harassment, and marriage equality is critical in your work with all clients, but it's especially important to understand yourself when working with gender care clients.

Sexual Orientation vs. Gender Expression

The concepts of sexual orientation and gender expression can be quite confusing to many people, including therapists. I believe this comes from stereotypes of gender norms. Gender isn't necessarily about sex. Part of our personal and self-expression does come out in a sexual arena, but we express our gender in many other ways that have nothing to do with sex. To be affirming of our clients, we have to recognize the differences between sexuality and gender.

Gender is an expression of characteristics. Historically in American culture, this has been defined by a "masculine/feminine" binary; however, there are countless ways that people express their gender. Therapists have to encourage clients to identify authentic gender expression that best fits, while recognizing this can vary greatly from person to person.

Sexual orientation is more about the attraction that people have for other people. This can be sexual, but it's not only sexual. It's also emotional, spiritual and even mental. Sexual orientation can also be about connection, and some of that connection results in sex.

Again, our culture creates schemas, which lead to stereotypes and binaries. It's in our nature to categorize, and we prefer to keep to as few gender and sexual orientation categories as possible. This leads to strict binaries such as "man/woman" and "gay/straight," but these limitations aren't based in reality. Sexual orientation and gender occur on a spectrum, and the expressive needs of people vary.

There is a wide array of sexual orientation identification for people who are transgender, gender queer, and gender non-binary. When some individuals begin to feel more open to express their gender, they might have a different point of view about their sexuality. Practicing authenticity might help these people further expand on their understanding of themselves, and perspectives on sexuality could be part of this process.

Therapists need to allow clients to establish their own goals. It's important to avoid suggesting identity issues that aren't present. Therapists can make the mistake of creating a sexual orientation issue when this isn't an issue for that client at all. For example, therapists will sometimes assign labels of "gay," "lesbian," and "straight" to a client who isn't identifying with them. Clients need the space to label themselves and to go without labels as well.

A Deeper Look at Gender, Sexual Orientation, and "Fetishization" in Cisgender Men Who Step Outside of Norms

There are few things that confuse therapists more than cisgender men wearing women's clothing. What does it mean when these men come in for therapy? It depends.

The most common misconception that I hear is also usually wrong. When a man wears women's clothing, a lot of therapists assume that he is gay, which may not be the case at all. The clothing we choose to wear doesn't dictate our sexual orientation. In fact, it doesn't dictate our gender identity either. Yet, people continue to confuse sexual orientation and gender expression all of the time.

Clients who identify as cisgender men are often treated with suspicion and judgment by their families in these situations. They can be treated with suspicion by therapists as well. Their self-identification is often put into doubt by both. We have rigid boundaries around men. In a heterosexual marriage, this situation can be very intimidating for a wife because people are wrongfully taught myths about sex and gender.

There are times when a man wearing women's clothing is sexual. For example, some men may wear women's clothing while masturbating. A man may also like the feeling of the clothing and find it arousing. In these situations, this may be something that the couple integrates into their relationship. It can also become a private, sexual behavior that the couple knows is occurring, yet they don't engage in it together.

There are times when wearing women's clothing isn't sexual at all. If it's the way the clothes look or feel that is pleasurable, it's very possible this is non-sexual. Our job is to help our clients find self-acceptance and personal understanding without feeding into bias.

When it's a couple seeking out our help, we have to help them process their boundaries and thoughts surrounding gender. The couple also has to understand their fears. As they process this information, they can determine whether this relationship is workable. I've found the *Gottman-Rapoport Conflict Blueprint* to be a useful tool for helping couples discuss this in a balanced way. This blueprint offers an opportunity for clients to share their stories in a non-shaming manner.

> There are times when behaviors are outside of cisgender norms because they are an expression of gender. This person may come to identify as transgender as more self-discovery occurs. Therapists must recognize that this isn't always the case. It's called a "journey" for a reason. Again, most people assume that they're cisgender. When therapy is a safe place, some clients do come to realize that they're actually on a gender spectrum that they hadn't previously realized.

Gender expression varies significantly from person to person. For our clients who are identifying authentic ways of expressing themselves, we have to respect the many different ways that people might do this. Be careful not to make broad assumptions about how gender expression should look in your clients' lives.

Those who identify with genders that are outside of the norms of our binary culture have likely contended with various forms of cultural and historical trauma. Thus, therapists really need specialized training and/or consultation with an expert in gender care to work with this group. Transgender and nonbinary individuals can experience high levels of discrimination, transphobia, hate, and abuse in their lifetimes. Therapy can be a very powerful resource for these individuals, as well as their families, but if therapists don't have adequate training, even the most well-intentioned person can cause a lot of harm.

Gender Pronouns and the Importance of Non-Binary Acceptance

By now you've read how extreme thinking can impact therapists and our clients. I've already talked about the impact of extreme thinking on sexual orientation. People also struggle with understanding the non-binary of gender as well. One of the primary ways through which we express our gender is through the use of pronouns.

For our clients, appropriate use of gender pronouns can be one of the most validating parts of their journey. At the same time, when the wrong pronoun is used, it can be shaming, invalidating, and painful. Using requested pronouns is extremely important for these clients.

These pronouns may not fit binaries. For example, rather than "he" or "she", "they" or "them" may feel the most authentic. How do you know which feels the most authentic to your client? You have to ask.

Sex-positive therapy requires a lot of mindfulness. Our minds can play tricks on us and lead us to use the wrong pronouns. The following steps can help you remain mindful and hold space for your clients. They can also help you circle back around when you screw up. Here is the advice that I give other therapists on how to avoid hurtful mistakes, while also rectifying situations where mistakes were made:

1. **Slow down.**
   Most mistakes happen when we move too fast. By taking your time, you're less likely to make assumptions that could be hurtful.

2. **The client is the expert.**

    To identify clients in the most authentic way, you have to ask. They will name the pronouns, labels, and non-labels that they want to use. It's the therapist's responsibility to utilize these labels and recognize that they might change.

3. **Own your mistakes.**

    If you misgender a client, use the wrong pronouns, or make a wrongful assumption about their sexual orientation, don't try to cover it up. By owning your mistake, you have a wonderful opportunity to build a great rapport with your client. If you attempt to cover it up, you'll lose an opportunity for your client to process their emotions around the mistake.

4. **Own your limitations in understanding.**

    As a sexuality expert, you can never know more than the person who is living in the experience. Embrace the vulnerability of asking questions when you don't know.

Transitioning

Some of the people who come into therapy for gender care are unsure of the direction that leads to authenticity. I've worked with many who need to process their situations in therapy before making decisions about hormone therapy (HT), gender marker changes on state identification, and surgery. Therapy can offer these clients a safe place to learn about themselves.

Sadly, therapists have been placed in the role of gate-keepers for gender transitions. Physicians and public entities regularly require a letter from at least one therapist before they agree to HT or surgery.

Although I see value in therapy for all clients, therapy shouldn't be used as a required step for HT. Please go to www.wpath.org to see the most current recommendations for physicians and therapists on transgender care. When clients are forced to participate in therapy, it can create anxiety and shame.

I've also seen this role get abused by therapists more than I would like to admit. There are therapists who have unnecessarily held clients hostage in therapy out of greed or out of a misunderstanding of the transitioning process. In these situations, the therapist avoids offering clarity about the requirements needed to get the required letter for HT or surgery. This is an abuse of power and it can make clients feel helpless when they're already in a state of high anxiety.

Therapists have to practice openness to help gender care clients with their process. When boundaries prevent them from writing a letter, the need to be clearly defined and a plan needs to be developed to address them. I recommend making it as transparent as creating a list and then having the client check in with you about their progress on this list. These steps need to be as concrete as possible. Providing such a list helps clients maintain hope and it builds trust by showing them that you're not trying to get in the way of their transition journey.

I also recommend that therapists help their gender care clients develop a timeline for their transition. A timeline helps clients identify their long-term goals of authenticity and gender expression. It also helps them identify smaller steps that need to happen to get there. This process also offers an opportunity to ask clients questions and provide education as needed. I always point out to clients that these goals will often change over time and this is only a current idea of their journey. I want them to know that they can change their journey or add to it as they walk into new arenas of self-discovery.

Clients can process this journey through an exercise that is similar to the Extremes Exercise that I discussed earlier. I want to point out that it's critical to ensure that there is an adequate therapeutic alliance before doing this. Again, gender care clients are often suspicious of the "gate-keeping" aspect of therapy. They often have a fear of being shamed by the therapist. By building a strong relationship, clients may be more inclined to openly explore their journey and insecurities with you.

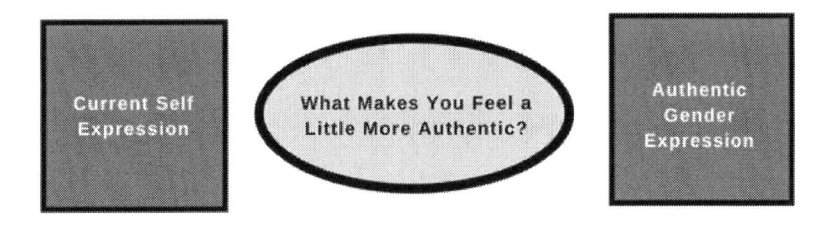

| Current Self Expression | What Makes You Feel a Little More Authentic? | Authentic Gender Expression |

"Passing," Shame, and How You Can Help

Passing is a term that reflects gender expression that fits within our culture's constructs of an identified gender. When people question our clients' gender, it can be a shaming experience for them. Gender care clients often feel safest when their gender isn't questioned by others.

I have to disclose my own personal bias on this issue. I believe the Passing expectation is often rooted in the shame that comes from a biased culture. Call it my rebellious nature, but part of me wants all transgender people to denounce this and feel free to show who they are without this fear. I don't want them to be bound to conforming to constructs that were set up by other groups of people.

> The truth is that this is my own cisgender bias. I don't personally know what it's like to travel on this gender journey. It's easy for me to say that Passing shouldn't matter, because I haven't had the experiences that transgender and non-conforming people regularly do. I can pontificate to them about my idealized perspective, but that isn't the world that these clients live in.
>
> I share this to provide an example of how bias can be rooted in good intentions. When we let cisgender biases influence our interactions with our clients, we can invalidate them. Notice that I don't rid myself of my bias in this scenario. I simply recognize it, own up to why I view the world in this way, and accept that my clients' perspectives will be different. This helps me respect my clients' journeys.
>
> The best way to facilitate discussions about Passing is to allow clients to identify their own needs. Even with increased self-acceptance, clients often feel that Passing is important to them. It's important that we respect and support this.

Basic Rules for Letters for Gender Care Clients

The gate-keeping role is often placed on the shoulders of therapists because letters are still required by a majority of physicians before they'll agree to HT or surgery. Here, I am naming some basic rules that can help protect our liability and our clients as well.

The following are rules for therapists when writing letters for gender care clients:

1. **If you refuse to write a letter, then you have to know why.**

   Some therapists won't offer reasons for denying these letters. Their vagueness appears mired in their desire to keep a client on their schedule, rather than actually advocating for their clients' needs. Sadly, I've had conversations with therapists who couldn't really articulate why they were refusing a letter. For example, I remember a therapist saying, "I just don't think they are ready." Therapists must be able to name concrete reasons behind their refusal, or refer the client to another affirming therapist.

2. **The client needs to know what they want and who they want to work with.**

   I've had an occasional client who wanted a letter and yet wasn't really sure why. They might describe wanting it just in case they "need to use it" later on. There is a professional liability that we have as therapists, which must be respected. Although I don't think these clients are intentionally trying to disrespect our liability, they're often unaware of this. In these situations, I've gently explained the boundary, so that clients can identify the reasons why they need a letter. I also require that they know what physician they're seeking out as well. Most clients are understanding of this boundary when it's explained.

3. **Clients need to have some awareness of the potential changes and side effects of the next step they're identifying on their journey.**

Most clients are aware of potential side effects of HT. Many of the side effects are desired (i.e. breast enlargement, voice changes, skin changes, etc.). Therapists can discuss some of these, but physicians are also responsible for educating their clients about this. We can help clients identify holes in their knowledge, while also helping them identify questions that they need to ask other providers.

4. **There must be no identifiable diagnoses that are currently preventing the client from making coherent, reality-based decisions.**

   Clients need to be oriented to person, place, and time. If they aren't, we need to put the letter on hold. More assessment is needed so that steps can be identified to work collaboratively with this client to get them on more stable ground.

5. **If you refuse a letter, give specific steps for the client to follow.**

   Several of our gender care clients have lived with feelings of hopelessness and helplessness. I would even say that this is true of a majority of these clients. Their ongoing gender transition is usually a place of hope if it keeps progressing. When we don't offer specific steps, we can crush a resourceful place of hope. Do the opposite. Identify and list the steps that need to be taken.

There are other important rules to consider when writing a letter. For more information about transitioning, every therapist who works with gender care should refer to the current version of the WPATH Standards of Care.

> **If You're LGBT Affirming, Then You Have to Include the "T"**
>
> I've noticed a sad trend in our field. Several therapists and treatment programs say that they're LGBT affirming or "friendly," yet they don't want to work with transgender clients. This can lead to an extremely shaming experience for transgender people. Imagine what it's like to become brave enough to reach out to a therapist, only to have that therapist deny you services because of your gender. Please don't carelessly use "LGBT" as a marketing strategy. If you use this acronym, you need to be prepared to accept transgender clients, or at least help them get the resources they need when they contact you.

Affirming Therapy for Gender Care Clients

Ongoing consultation and training are essential elements to providing quality services to transgender and gender non-binary individuals. I believe that most therapists who work with gender care clients benefit from specific training, supervision, and consultation. In the meantime, there are some basic rules you can follow to help ensure that you're offering affirming services to your clients. Here are basic rules for therapists who offer affirming services for gender care clients:

- Don't assign pronouns. Allow clients to assign them. Clients might prefer pronouns that you're not accustomed to using.
- Focus on humanness and connection.
- Don't say you understand when you don't.
- Genitalia isn't your business unless the client wants to talk about this.
- Avoid making assumptions about sexual orientation.

- Support their transition journey as they define it.
- If a letter is required, name the steps that are needed to get one written for them.
- Know your own rigid biases about gender.

Sexual Compulsivity in Transgender or Gender Non-Binary Individuals

For some individuals who are dealing with gender dysphoria, compulsive numbing can become a coping mechanism. There are times when compulsive sexual behaviors can be linked to sexual and gender expression. Clients shouldn't be pushed into "abstaining" from gender expressive behaviors. Some will label their own expressive needs as an addictive pattern.

Therapists should work with clients to help them identify when their behaviors are compulsive and/or numbing. It's important to identify some of the elements that trigger a desire to numb. This desire often reflects those interpersonal struggles with disconnection and shame that I discussed earlier. Therapists also have to help clients discover balanced ways of expressing gender and sexuality as they grow into more self-acceptance.

Some people numb with pornography. Mindfulness can help clients become more in touch with their bodies by enhancing the body-mind connection. Numbing is typically shame-based. There is so much social pressure to conform to something other than who that person is.

Therapists need to handle mindfulness work delicately and patiently. Because this type of therapeutic work can be so intense, less is more when working with a population that deals with such a high level of societal shame. Using too much mindfulness therapy too early may push your clients into an emotional area that they aren't ready to handle. Remember, numbing is a coping mechanism. Therefore, it's important to be patient with your clients and give them space so they can build a tolerance to the vulnerability of authentically expressing themselves.

Clients who are experiencing gender dysphoria can deal with high levels of traumatic organization. One way of coping with shame, anxiety, fear of acceptance, and loss is to compartmentalize. Our clients often find it difficult to understand gender dysphoria because of emotional compartmentalization. Congruency is the goal for everyone, but going back into the closet and returning to massive denial can be tempting for some clients. Therapy should include gentle mindfulness work to help with levels of congruency and self-identification. When clients do head back into the closet, therapists need to practice patience and remain gentle.

As part of transitioning, clients have to identify what expression will look like to them. Expression can include wearing different clothes, voice changes, mannerisms, and voice tone. Therapists can offer information about possible ways of self-expression, but clients have to identify what feels most authentic.

When the client and therapist identify numbing patterns, validation of shame and the fear of vulnerability can help clients. Numbing is an understandable coping mechanism to respond to a culture that is rigid in its thinking about gender. Creating a space of understanding helps clients make sense of their behavior. With increased validation and shame resilience, numbing often becomes less necessary.

There are times when this numbing can transform into compulsive behavior. Standard exercises and assessments must be handled with extreme caution. Clients in this group may over-label their gender expressive needs as an addiction. The cisgender normalization of our society can make it easy for clients to misidentify and mislabel themselves. For example, a person might engage in cross-dressing and label this as a behavior problem. However, they may come to realize that this is a part of their congruent need for expression. The dividing line often reflects a difference between connection and disconnection. Therapists can hold space for clients to help them reconnect with friends, community, and sometimes family.

Suicide Prevention in the LGBTQ Community

Suicide risk is higher among LGBTQ individuals. Some research shows that up to 10% of LGBTQ individuals have attempted suicide in their lifetimes. Even more staggering, other research suggests that up to 40% of transgender people have attempted suicide in their lifetimes. People in this community regularly deal with isolation, abuse, and shame. Cultural issues can lead to increased stress, which also increases the risk for suicidal ideation. Others may have been assaulted, kicked out of their homes, or shunned by their communities and families.

Apart from these obvious issues, there are more subtle problems that people in this group have to contend with as well. Society normalizes heterosexuality and cisgender expression. These cultural structures send messages to LGBTQ adults, and especially adolescents and children that they're different and even inferior.

Shame, depression, and anxiety are also common issues for members of these groups. Therefore, suicide prevention must always be a part of counseling or therapy for LGBTQ clients. Some clients only require a quick assessment to assure their safety. Others will require in-depth safety planning and may even require a referral to a higher level of care.

During any coming-out process, regular check-ins with clients are needed to ensure that there is no suicidal ideation. Adolescent and child clients are even more at risk. They're particularly vulnerable to potential problems with bullying and family dynamics when dealing with their sexual orientation or gender. Therefore, we must remain aware of the potential risk of suicide and be prepared to intervene as needed.

4

Considerations for Kink, BDSM, and "Fetishes"

Kink, BDSM, and "fetishes" are also very vulnerable to being inappropriately labeled as sex addictions. Our culture tends to pathologize these behaviors, desires, and subcultures. Psychotherapists and counselors are at risk of buying into these cultural norms. Pathologizing can lead to increased levels of shame, and those who are discussed in this chapter are at a high risk of being misunderstood.

In this chapter, I will discuss some of the problems and relationship issues that can lead clients to come into our therapy offices. Similar to other groups I've discussed in this book, shame is often an undertone of these problems. I will also discuss considerations that you need to keep in mind in order to separate compulsive behavior from shame-based reactivity. Of course, we'll be discussing consent and boundaries as well.

This chapter isn't to serve as an overall competency training for kink and BDSM. Therapists need training and/or consultation to offer the best care to these clients. Instead, I want you to view this chapter as a potential starting point. I will be naming various biases later in this chapter. I will also be discussing education options that you can consider to help you avoid over-pathologizing. I hope your journey of learning about non-traditional desire and arousal will go well beyond this chapter.

The Shame in Labels and What to Consider

"Distress" is one of the most common symptoms of any diagnosis in the DSM; however, distress isn't necessarily a sign of a person's dysfunction. This can be a response to broader social prejudices. Distress is more often an outcome of cultural stigmas than a problematic "symptom" of kink, BDSM, and "fetishes."

Our culture has established noteworthy lines of "normal" vs. "abnormal" that it assigns to sexual behaviors, desire, and fantasies. A lot of this is based in our culture and history. Anything perceived as abnormal by our culture can be given a negative label and stigmatized. There is a common assumption that kink is an "alternative" lifestyle that only a rare few engage in. These assumptions, along with the vagueness of the symptom of distress, can lead to pathologizing behavior, desire, and play when they don't require diagnosing at all.

Why is "Fetish" in Quotes?

I have an overall issue with the word fetish because I believe that it has a negative connotation. "Fetish" is a word that is often used to describe the abnormal. This could be related to the history of the word being used in the DSM. When people think of the diagnoses listed in the DSM, they typically see these labels as a list of negative, problematic symptoms.

That being said, "fetish" is a recognizable word. In this book, you will notice that I put the word in quotes. I did this to specify that I appreciate and respect that this is a label. I also respect the implications that this label may have on people. There are many things that can be described as "fetishes" that go well beyond what I could name in this book. I don't pretend that one word can summarize the dynamics of every arousal, desire, behavior, and fantasy that could be categorized under this word. At the same time, using this word helps me simplify significant points in this book.

I don't want my use of this word to take away from the importance of mindfully remaining aware of the potential consequences of using this label. Therefore, by putting "fetish" in quotations, I hope it serves as a reminder of the power of this label. I also hope it reminds you of how important it is to discuss labels with your clients to identify what best fits them.

Several have high levels of shame about their non-traditional desires, fantasies, and arousal. This is especially true of the clients who come into our office. It's true of all of the groups discussed in this book. Clients have to unpack what authenticity is to them, as well as when they're responding to shame.

Sadly, our clients often know that there are biases in the therapy community about kink, BDSM, and "fetishes." They have a right to be cautious. Many therapists struggle with judgment about these communities. These biases can be blatant or subtle. Again, I'm not saying that you shouldn't have any biases because I don't believe that is realistic. In fact, cultural competency is about recognizing your own biases, so that you can work through them to help your clients rather than hinder their progress.

All clients are aware that therapists may view them as "unhealthy." Psychology has a long, painful history of abusing, shaming, and isolating people who are dealing with mental health issues. Just seeing a therapist can kick up these remnants of shame. Sex inherently comes with its own level of shame. This isn't even considering negative feelings that come with judgments about taboo behaviors and desires. If you add all of this to the shame that people experience about therapy, of course there will be distress in our clients.

I'm not saying that the DSM and diagnoses hold no value. Instead, I'm pointing out the power we hold with the labels that we use. Clients will judge themselves, and therapists will often judge them as well. Distress is an understandable, cultural response to the therapeutic process. I especially believe it's understandable for the clients we're discussing in this chapter.

All of these dynamics can prevent clients from accepting and sharing their desires, fantasies, and "fetishes." Clients may avoid communicating these things with their partners. This can lead to relationship problems, secrets, and many other personal problems. Shame and distress can also bring clients into therapy for sexual addiction. Working with these clients is another balancing act for therapists. In clients' lives and relationships, congruency, authenticity, and boundaries are always at the center of the therapeutic process.

There is a myth that sexual desire can be changed when others consider it "unhealthy." There is no evidence that therapy can eliminate any sexual desire or arousal. This is true of those who are discussed in this chapter as well. Clients will have to make personal decisions about how they express their desires, but they aren't going to erase them.

Relationships, Boundaries, and Self-Expression

People who come into therapy with concerns regarding their non-traditional arousal or desire are often in relationships. In fact, fear of losing these relationships can bring these clients into therapy. In these situations, it's common for clients to misunderstand kink, "fetishes," or BDSM. Misconceptions about a particular behavior, a sexual mismatch, cheating and infidelity, and shame are common reasons that clients seek out our help. There are also some clients who seek out a therapist for concerns about sexual compulsivity.

I've worked with several clients over the years who were at a high risk of ignoring their needs to save their relationships. Some have wanted to compartmentalize their needs. This can lead to future resentment or relationship issues. To save relationships, some clients who are interested in kink and BDSM label themselves as sex addicts. Some of them are dealing with compulsive sexual behavior, but many of are not.

Therapy has to be a safe place for these clients. Therapists have to be open and ask gentle probing questions. This helps clients identify what they want to remain in fantasy and what they need in their reality. It takes a lot of trust for clients to be open about desires when they can be considered taboo. While opening these doors, clients are often responding to society's judgments of what is considered abnormal. Therefore, it's common that they struggle with self-acceptance.

In my experience, members of the groups discussed in this chapter can experience personal confusion that is similar to that which I discussed with the LGBTQ community. People can downplay their desires and fantasies when they don't fit traditional cultural norms. This confusion can come from a lack of self-acceptance. Non-traditional desire is rarely depicted in popular culture. Movies and books such as the *50 Shades of Grey* series have brought kink into the mainstream. Like many other early attempts at mainstreaming, this comes with many flaws. Popular culture usually utilizes stereotypes in its depictions of various groups. *50 Shades of Grey* was no exception to utilizing stereotypes. For example, in the *50 Shades* plotline, kink is depicted as if it's something that always comes from a place of trauma.

These depictions can be beneficial because they show interest in what has otherwise been considered taboo. At the same time, they can create even more confusion. For example, in an overly romantic sense, the *50 Shades* series made it seem like someone who has BDSM needs requires rescuing. I know that these are just movies and it is make-believe; however, for people who have few accurate representations of themselves in popular culture, confusion about themselves can be very common.

Whether clients have a problem with sexual compulsivity or not, they often experience incongruence regarding love, relationships, trust, and commitment. Our clients who are in relationships often have layers of problems with communication and connection. Kink, BDSM, and "fetishes" are often blamed for these problems. This blame can promote incongruence and confusion in someone who is has kinky or "fetishistic" desires. Therapy can help with this process.

Deepening an Understanding of Boundaries

Everyone should have negotiable and non-negotiable boundaries. Helping clients deepen their understanding of their boundaries is critical to maintaining a relationship. When people gain a better understanding, they're more likely to listen, empathize with one another, and work together on what is negotiable.

In therapy, I usually start by helping the people in the relationship share their assumptions about needs, beliefs about the other person, and expectations from the other person. So often, these assumptions are wrong. This allows them to clarify these assumptions with each other. Doing this can offer insight into the fears, vulnerabilities, and insecurities of everyone in the relationship. It can also help to develop an understanding of relationship dreams and goals. All of this information can increase empathy. It also increases trust. Trust takes a hit in any relationship that has a lot of misunderstanding.

It's important to encourage our clients to deepen their personal understanding of their feelings because they often struggle to identify their boundaries. This understanding about themselves can help establish their lines of comfort.

Sometimes, when people increase trust and empathy in the relationship, non-negotiable boundaries may shift. People may be willing to step into new arenas, while some boundaries will always remain non-negotiable. Connection can still improve, even when couples agree to not engage in certain behaviors. It can be empowering to learn how to talk about these boundaries rather than tuck them away and shut them down.

Therapists have a responsibility to help their clients establish boundaries and open communication in their relationships. Many people are surprised by how much acceptance they get from their partners when they're open, despite the shame that they've felt. Open dialogue helps people in the relationship discuss what they're going to do with this information as it's more out in the open.

Not Assuming that Monogamy is the Answer

When there is acceptance of non-traditional desires and needs, some of our clients conclude that non-monogamy might work for them. There is a myth that non-monogamy inherently diminishes the primary relationship, but for some, it can even enhance it. When there are solid boundaries and agreements, non-monogamy is a possibility.

It's important to note that non-monogamy isn't for everyone. Therapists shouldn't push their clients into this. At the same time, we can ask them questions to see how they feel about this possibility. Most couples haven't even considered this possibility before being asked about it.

Whether a couple wants this in their relationship or not, asking about consensual non-monogamy can help them process relationship goals. Promoting this discussion also encourages couples to identify their overall relationship goals. This can bring them closer together in a way that promotes open dialogue. This also helps to prevent resentment.

If the couple does decide to open up their relationship, they can process ground rules. For help with these boundaries, please refer to

Chapter 6, which focuses on consensual non-monogamy in relationships.

The Need for Sexual Attitudes Reassessment (SAR)

The Sexual Attitudes Reassessment (SAR) course is extremely important for therapists who work with kink, BDSM and non-traditional behavior or arousal. This course is a required part of the certification process to become an AASECT Certified Sex Therapist. This course helps therapists process their feelings, biases, and prejudices about non-traditional desire and sex, while participating in an engaging process.

This group, like many of those discussed in this book, can be sensitive to therapist bias and judgment. Therapists have to be aware of their levels of comfort and discomfort. Therapists often overestimate their level of acceptance. Even when they believe they're accepting of their clients, they can still project subtle elements of unacceptance. SAR courses can help therapists identify these subtleties.

When participating in the SAR course, therapists come face-to-face with images, scenes, and considerations for various sexual relationships, orientations, arousal, and expressions. They're allowed to process their perceptions and attitudes about several types of sexual expression, desire, orientation, etc. Those who may have previously struggled with a lack of understanding about non-traditional sexual expression can identify their personal struggle with acceptance. This can be very challenging, but I highly recommend it for any therapist who wants to work with these groups.

The Dynamics of Holding Space for Kink, BDSM, and Fetishes

Unfortunately, many therapists continue to make the mistake of labeling non-traditional behaviors as an addiction. Pain, power dynamics, certain types of play, and sexual aids are often over-pathologized as problems. Therapists have to respect that these elements are likely to remain somewhere in the template of attraction, desire, or eroticism for this person. It's also important to be non-shaming while people explore self-expression.

Our field has a long history of labeling and even psychoanalyzing kink, BDSM, and "fetishes" as disorders. This comes from the illusion that we can retrace the origins of our arousal and change it. There is little consistent evidence that this can be accomplished. There is also no clear evidence that retracing this information is needed. It comes from a biased perspective that promotes the pathologizing of non-traditional expression.

I'm not suggesting that clients should never explore their sexual development. In fact, developmental information can be helpful for our clients as they learn more about themselves. Instead, I'm saying that therapists need to be cautious of overinterpreting the meaning of behavior, desire, and arousal. Although some people may come to their own understanding of their sexual development, this isn't an exact science. Developmental stories and their meaning vary greatly from person to person.

Shame and the Desire for Arousal Extinction

The therapy field has the potential to increase shame for all of the vulnerable groups in this book. Later in this book, I will be talking about the "expert-mania" that is taking over our field. Popular psychology has taught many potential clients that they need to seek out therapists because they are experts.

A strong sense of expertise can lead therapists to overestimate their ability to change people. Clients who are interested in kink, BDSM, and "fetishes" are at a high risk of shame. When therapists over-embrace their expert status and clients are struggling with shame, a dangerous outcome becomes more likely.

When shame and anxiety are high, clients sometimes come into therapy with a desire to "wipe out" non-traditional arousal, desires, etc. They will look for "experts" who believe in this "wipe-out" process. Sadly, these therapists aren't hard to find. I liken them to therapists who offer SOCE to LGBTQ clients; however, therapists who claim to be able to erase kink, BDSM, and "fetishes" are more widely accepted than those who offer SOCE. Sadly, they don't have to disguise their intentions at all.

I can still recall one particularly painful example of this expert-shame dynamic. I had a client who was told that Eye Movement Desensitization and Reprocessing (EMDR) could help "wipe out" his attraction to an object. As a therapist who is trained in EMDR, I found this appalling. There is no evidence that EMDR has any efficacy in erasing sexual desire. This client had a lot of shame about his erotic desire. Thus, when a therapist offered him an opportunity to rid himself of this, he jumped at the chance. When it didn't work, he blamed himself.

Shame played an integral part in this case. When I worked with him, I helped this client build shame resilience. We had to do a lot of therapeutic work about his past therapy experiences and the harm that was caused. As he became more resilient to shame, he found a way to increase his sense of what he wanted in his life. Prior to working with me, he struggled with the impulse to secretly watch others. In therapy, he came to realize that this was related to shame. After working on negative emotions, authenticity, and self-acceptance, the behavior of watching others stopped.

Out of our therapeutic desire to help, we risk playing the role of experts in a way that is unrealistic and harmful. I believe that using therapy to "eradicate" non-traditional desire is a boundary violation that is based in moral superiority and power. When therapists try to eradicate kink, BDSM, and "fetishes," they're putting their values system and beliefs onto their clients. The clients are the ones who pay the price.

People in these groups often hold a lot of shame, which prevents them from sharing their desires with their partner(s). They're likely to experience distress. This sometimes reaches a point of maladaptive coping, which has the potential to become out of control and even reach a point of compulsivity. I'll be discussing compulsivity later in this chapter.

I encourage a therapeutic environment that revolves around self-acceptance. Many of my clients have struggled with over-identification with their arousal and desire. Again, arousal and desire are unlikely to disappear. There are several aspects to all people, and arousal and desire are only a part of the picture. When there is incongruency with arousal, there is a greater risk of it becoming an obsessive element of a person's life. I believe that a lack of self-acceptance can create an obsession with arousal and desire, because it requires a lot of energy to compartmentalize these things. Openness in therapy can prompt decompartmentalization that helps bring balance back into our clients' lives.

For clients who haven't yet shared their desires with their partner(s), the relationship can be a source of distress. There is often anxiety about the vulnerability of exposing this information. In situations where there hasn't been betrayal in the relationship, clients will often find partners who are supportive. This doesn't mean that all relationships can welcome kink, BDSM, and "fetish" elements, but some of them are able to after they engage in open dialogue and negotiations.

When there are betrayals in our clients' relationships, therapists have to remain understanding of the cultural dynamics here as well. When it comes to kink, BDSM, and "fetishes," some of our clients enter into marriage, without any knowledge of this part of themselves. Others recognize these things about themselves, but believed that this would just remain private. Then there are those who entered into relationships thinking that these desires would change and even evaporate over time. This is often because kink, BDSM, and "fetishes" don't fit into the traditional education that our clients receive about relationships, sex, and desire. Therefore, people are often unaware of these parts of who they are.

We have a responsibility to offer compassionate care for our clients who are hurt partners, who have also experienced betrayal from cheating. There are partners who will be fearful of kink, BDSM, and "fetish" based desires. Some of them might project the pain they have experienced from betrayal onto desires of kink, BDSM, and "fetishes." They might view discussions about this topic as threatening as well. It's critical to show partners empathy, without shaming them for their fears and pain.

Therapists also have to be understanding of the reasons that clients may not be forthcoming at the beginning of therapy about kink, BDSM, and "fetishes." It's true that dishonesty and withholding of information are common in addicts. Lacking trust is also common for people who have desires that are outside of sociocultural norms. Therefore, "lies of omission" aren't great signs of an addiction when working with vulnerable groups. Other corroborating evidence is important as well.

Not all clients will come into therapy due to relationship problems. Some will have very accepting partners and want to negotiate new elements into their relationships. Therapy can serve as a place for open dialogue and understanding. It can also be a great place for clients to build and establish boundaries.

I've also worked with clients from this group who avoid relationships. In these situations, they have generally sought out my help because of their fear of rejection in potential connections. In my experience, these clients often want relationships, but need to work on their shame resilience. When they increase their tolerance to shame, they're more likely to take chances on establishing relationships.

Infidelity in Kink, BDSM, and "Fetishes"

As you have read before, shame is a major predictor of secrecy, lying, and cheating. Shame is often connected to a person's cultural experiences. For those who would like to add elements of kink or BDSM to their relationships, shame can influence individuals and relationships. This is also true of people who have desire and arousal that has been historically classified as "fetishes."

There are more open discussions of desire and arousal than ever before in our society. Unfortunately, I believe that the increased openness is actually used as a punchline to jokes in our media, rather than used to promote true, fair, and open conversations. In these portrayals, kink, BDSM, and "fetishes" are still unfairly linked to shaming theories of perversion. They're often also correlated with psychological damage. These portrayals send a message that people need to be ashamed of this part of who they are and that they should keep it a secret.

Shame doesn't erase cheating or dishonesty. Nor does it erase the heartbreak and trauma that come from betrayal, but it's important to recognize that shame does increase the risk of lying and cheating. Those who live with non-traditional desires regularly feel as though their partners could never accept them, which influences their openness. Honesty is always a choice, yet secrecy can be understandable when we view it through an empathetic lens.

Is Non-Traditional Arousal an Orientation?

This question is part of an ongoing, controversial debate. It has been my clinical experience that sexual desire and arousal come in all forms. I've yet to see a case where non-traditional desire has completely disappeared from a client. Many of our clients have already tried to rid themselves of shameful desire and fantasy before they come into our offices. Even those who are struggling with sexual boundaries and compulsive sexual behavior will usually report that the desire remains after therapy. Most evidence shows that arousal itself won't entirely disappear.

> Therefore, although controversial, my experiences have led me to believe that desire is an unchangeable orientation. Desire may undulate and shape-shift over time. There are situations where people identify desire and attraction that wasn't previously there. I've seen no evidence that this is changeable by an external force like therapy. Therefore, we have to help our clients process this, identify their needs and wants, and find ways of self-acceptance that reflect boundaries and personal values.

When many of these clients reflect on cheating behavior, they come to identify that they felt "trapped" or "constrained" by the initial agreement of the relationship. They didn't know how to go about opening up a dialogue. This doesn't justify cheating, but it can help us understand the situation, which can also help us as therapists.

Other clients may have a history of better self-awareness. They recognize their non-traditional arousal or desire in their lives, but these clients are at a risk of thinking that desire will just go away. Therefore, it seems unnecessary to address it in their relationship. These clients might also feel that they're experiencing something that should remain in the fantasy realm; however, things can change as a relationship grows and more negotiations may take place over time.

Again, infidelity isn't the same as addiction. There are times when cheating behavior may be compulsive. Other times, the behavior may reflect the shame that we've talked so much about. There are situations where shameful secrecy and compulsive behavior will overlap as well.

For those relationships that have experienced an affair, they can no longer enjoy the luxuries of assumptions. I prefer that more people talk openly about all aspects of their lives before betrayal occurs, but the majority of people who come to therapy don't have a history of this. Clients often continue to avoid talking openly, even after an affair or infidelity.

It's common for our clients to want to return to silence after conversations about boundaries have been opened up. Even in their relationships, avoidance of difficult topics can keep people comfortable. It helps people avoid the feeling of vulnerability that comes with difficult conversations. These people are often resistant to talking about desire, fearing that the outcome will be negative. Therapy can encourage them to step into these discussions.

It's important to remember that there will likely be a low tolerance to these conversations immediately after the discovery of an affair. When there is increased consistency and trust in the relationship, patience and understanding will increase over time. It's important to assess this tolerance regularly to determine how much we can push clients to step into this vulnerability zone.

How Trauma Therapy Can Help Rather than Hinder

Trauma work is important when working with non-traditional behaviors and arousal, but not necessarily for the reasons that you might think. Although several of these clients might want to work on past issues, we shouldn't assume that healing wounds from their pasts will "cure" desires in the present. There is a myth that trauma work can erase desire. Desire won't completely change for most.

Some of our clients will try to remain within their current relationship boundaries.

It has been my experience that trauma work can benefit clients who are at risk of cultural and traumatic shame. The clients discussed in this chapter are at a high risk of experiencing this. Many of my clients have had sociocultural experiences that have led to trauma. When they have problematic symptoms, they can often be linked to these experiences or the residual shame that comes from these experiences. As traumatic wounds are validated, self-acceptance can grow and the wounds can then heal.

Heavy compartmentalization is one of the most common hallmarks of trauma that I've seen in clients. When people believe that they can't be authentic, they compartmentalize who they are. When they do this, they live up to someone else's perception of them in one arena, and participate in other behaviors in another. This can set a foundation for addictive behavior.

Whether an addiction exists or not, shame resiliency therapy, combined with trauma work can be extremely beneficial to clients in this group. As clients increase their personal understanding, they become better able to communicate their needs, talk more openly with partners, and develop new ways of negotiating.

Building a Foundation with Trust

It's sad that so many people are consumed with shame that they won't open up with their partners. When people are open, partners are often much more accepting than was previously anticipated. Unfortunately, this opportunity for openness wasn't given to the majority of the people with whom we work.

Betrayal often buries openness and understanding. When people are betrayed, it's difficult for them to hear and understand the shame of their partners. As partners heal, understanding grows and more discussions about desires and needs can take place. People are also better able to process their boundaries as they heal from betrayal. This is usually after levels of trust are rebuilt and both have worked on their individual healing.

It's Not the Partner's Fault

Dishonesty, fear, shame, and cheating aren't the partner's fault. Although it seems like this should go without saying, partners can be blamed for these behaviors in therapy sessions. Some therapists accuse partners of being controlling, manipulative, and abusive.

I believe that sexism is a major influence on these perceptions. Women partners are more likely to receive negative labels than men, especially when they establish boundaries in their relationships. In fact, I've even heard therapists blame women partners for the cheating and lying of the other person.

I know I've already shared a lot of information about shame. It's important to help clients with shame resilience. It's also important to avoid placing the shame of one partner onto the shoulders of the other. Shame doesn't erase the painful experiences of the partner.

I also know that some therapists have shamed hurt partners in the name of being labeled as sex positive. Some therapists want to be kink-aware and affirming, but they do this at the expense of the partner. By shaming and blaming a partner for their boundaries, therapists can co-conspire with a gaslighting process.

Again, there is a balance in this work. It's important to avoid taking sides. It's important to help each individual define personal

> values and boundaries. We also have to help them come together and determine their relationship goals and boundaries.

As trust builds and these old wounds heal, it becomes easier to negotiate in relationships. I've found that clients often struggle with separating addictive/compulsive behavior from healthy, non-traditional desire, kink, and BDSM. In the situations that we work with, they can view these elements as a threat to their relationship. Therapists have to offer a balance between allowing partners to find non-shaming ways of sharing their concerns and feelings, while also promoting increased openness. In time, the couple can learn how to discuss these feelings and negotiate in a way that makes the most sense to them.

The Lines of Compulsivity

Although kink, BDSM, and "fetishes" aren't usually sexually compulsive, there are times when behavior patterns can become compulsive or obsessive. It's important to note that when clients step into this territory, it doesn't erase their needs and desires. Therefore, there are still open discussions and negotiations to be had in the future. Our job isn't to favor either side in this process, but to help the couple negotiate.

Compulsivity is identified by repeated behavior that causes distress. This ongoing behavior is combined with continued consequences. These consequences can vary from personal to relational to occupational. The person will usually express that they don't want to engage in the behavior, yet end up engaging in it again anyway.

It's important to note that many clients in this group will label their behavior as compulsive. They may have mixed feelings about their behavior. Clients can also have contradictory thoughts that say they shouldn't engage in this, yet desire to continue to engage in it. Part of the therapy process includes helping clients identify this type of compartmentalization and incongruency when it occurs.

Dissociation

A common collateral hallmark that I've seen in clients who are genuinely dealing with compulsivity is dissociation. I've had clients who literally told me that they suddenly became aware of the pain they were experiencing during the actual experience. Similarly, I've also had clients discuss moments where they became aware that they didn't want to participate in the behavior anymore, yet they continued to engage in it anyway.

There's another type of dissociative experience that doesn't revolve around the behavior. Some may not be addicted to the behavior itself, as much as they might be addicted to a person. Some people will override their boundaries and engage in a behavior out of fear. This can come from a fear of loss or a fear of being alone. It could even be from a fear of the other person.

Dissociation by itself doesn't make the behavior addictive or compulsive. When I do hear that this is occurring, I monitor for compulsivity. I also monitor for trauma. This helps me conceptualize questions that I will ask my clients, as well as interventions that I might try.

Boundary Violations and a Loss of Control

All of us need to have boundaries in our relationships. If we're being honest, most of us would sexually step outside these boundaries in our peak fantasies. Relationships are full of boundaries and negotiations. Some desires won't fit within the boundaries of some of our clients' relationships.

Clients who struggle with compulsivity often have a desire for relationship boundaries that they also ignore. This can become confusing for therapists, but also family members. In compulsive situations, people may continue to engage in behaviors that step outside these boundaries. They can even get to a space where they can't control their behavior patterns.

Relationships are also filled with decisions. People sometimes make rash decisions about sex. This is why it's important to remember that a single episode of mindlessness isn't an addiction. Addiction is more pervasive. Addiction involves multiple mindless experiences and behaviors. This process happens over and over again. It's not an isolated episode of numbing. It involves repeated numbing without a lot of awareness of how or why this keeps happening.

Preoccupied Obsession

There are those who struggle with preoccupation. Fantasizing is something that is normal and common. We all have sexual fantasies. For some, these fantasies can become obsessive. In these situations, a person might isolate and avoid others. They might cognitively obsess about their fantasies in a way that becomes all-consuming and exhausting.

Of course, we all think about sex differently. It's not a problem to think about sex, fantasy or desire; however, some can be so preoccupied that they neglect other elements of their lives. In these situations, they might ignore families and relationships. They can become overly distracted at work. There are several other examples of consequences that can come from obsession and compulsivity. What examples have you seen in your work with your clients?

> **Ongoing Self-Discovery in Recovery**
>
> Clients need time to explore who they are. Even when there is compulsivity, clients often want to add new elements into their lives and relationships. Therapy can be that open place where clients can explore this.
>
> Some therapists make the mistake of assuming that a client could never add these kinky elements to their lives, due to past compulsivity. But like other process addictions, complete abstinence from behaviors isn't always needed or even possible. We have to help clients explore their needs with openness, balance, and mindfulness.
>
> When clients gain confidence in themselves, they become better able to explore their needs. I regularly ask clients to describe their "must-haves" in their relationships. This doesn't necessarily mean that they have to immediately leave their relationship if they're with a partner who can't offer these "must-haves." Rather, it means that they have to process these needs with their partner in an open manner to determine what the next step might be.

Sex-Positive Considerations for Kink, "Fetishes," and BDSM

How will you respond if you're working with someone who has desire or arousal that is non-traditional? What if your client tells you that they're aroused by pain, particular objects or domination or submission? Would you believe that this was related to past abuse and that it's unhealthy?

Therapists often think that they can hide their true feelings. They think they can avoid shaming their clients. In my experience, most people in this group who come to therapy are incredibly sensitive of the judgment of others. It doesn't have to be blatantly said for them to pick up on it either.

While some people might choose to withhold information about themselves, there are others who will be more open with you in therapy. Almost all of our clients will be looking for cues of acceptance. However, the clients who are discussed in this chapter may look for these cues even more. When there is a sociocultural history of judgment and shame, people learn pretty quickly how to identify judgmental cues from others. These experiences make our clients keenly aware of when we're judging them in therapy as well.

You have to be aware of your judgments and feelings surrounding kink, BDSM, and "fetishes." There is no way to anticipate each and every type of arousal, need, and orientation that will come to your office. So, anticipating some of your boundaries and limitations is helpful. Recognizing this about yourself can prevent you from inadvertently shaming your clients.

How can you prepare yourself for these situations in therapy? It can be helpful to take a SAR class or a specific sex therapy course in working with these groups. These courses help you come to terms with your judgments. Without this exposure, it's difficult to recognize how you will feel in these situations.

I know I've said this before, but because it's so common, I'm going to repeat it here. There is a lot of harm that can come from over-estimating your open-mindedness and cultural competency. All of us therapists are vulnerable to this. I recommend that you know and anticipate how you feel about "fetishes," pain, and domination at the very least. Awareness and caution will help you identify your limitations and times when you need to refer to someone who is more affirming. If you feel as though nothing bothers you, then you need to look deeper. It's very possible that you're over-estimating or denying your boundaries, which means that you're more likely to harm or shame your clients without even knowing it.

You might not be aware of your discomfort with certain things until you come into contact with a client who crosses your boundaries. In situations like this, you'll need to identify whether you'll be comfortable enough to build trust in the therapeutic setting. I recommend that you discuss your boundaries with a colleague who will be honest with you about how uncomfortable you sound. This can help you gauge whether you can continue your work with this client or if you need someone who is more specialized in it.

There is no shame in needing to refer a client. No therapist is equipped to work with every person who walks through the door. Know where these lines are for you. This will protect your clients, but it will protect you from liability issues as well.

Supervision and clinical consultation are also important aspects of working with vulnerable groups. Consultation is a place where your colleagues can ask you challenging questions about your boundaries and limitations. You can identify underlying judgments and work through them accordingly. It can also help you fine-tune your knowledge and language skills, so that you know when you're unintentionally shaming your clients.

Looking at Your Biases

I want you to view the act of working with non-traditional sexuality as another type of cultural competency. We have a responsibility to understand the culture that impacts our clients. We also have a responsibility to understand ourselves as well. Take a look at the biases below and see how they might reflect your beliefs. Again, if done correctly, this will be uncomfortable, but you'll learn about yourself in the process.

Here are some common therapist biases about the groups discussed in this chapter:

- "Fetishes," BDSM, and kink are a response to trauma.
- This behavior is unhealthy.
- BDSM and kink are always related to childhood abuse.
- These needs are dysfunctional.
- Kink is a rare alternative lifestyle.
- Desires and needs in these groups are abusive.
- These clients don't know what they actually want.
- The outward expression of kink, "fetishes," and BDSM is dirty or disgusting.

These aren't the only biases that you might have. It's important to know what yours are before you start this work. If these don't reflect your beliefs, I encourage you to look deeper for the biases that you have. Knowing this can help you take your time and intervene with potential shame before it even takes place.

Clients' Exploration of Kink

When clients reach a place of healthy boundaries and solid relationship agreements, they might be interested in exploring kink. Some clients will want to explore this in the community, while others will want this to be more private. Therapists can play a supportive role in this part of their clients' journeys.

Local kink gatherings can be a useful way of exploring. "Munches" are one type of gathering that is a good place for newcomers to start. Most cities have sporadic, but regular events that take place as well. People who attend are welcome to directly engage, but they can also observe where open viewing is allowed at the gathering.

Interacting with community-based events provides several benefits. Clients can meet like-minded people. They might also find partners who are more likely to be accepting. They can explore their fantasies and desires. Last, but not least, they can get support while they're going through their journey towards self-expression. Although therapy can help with this, having accepting peers can be invaluable.

There is also a variety of literature, courses, and online forums that people can engage in as well. Some of these forums offer a little more anonymity for clients who aren't ready to explore this with other people in more public settings. Several sex educators offer kink aware education that is open to the community. The information that these resources offers can help people learn about themselves, while considering possibilities to explore.

When working with clients who have a history of compulsivity, it's important to help them remain mindful. It's essential that they work to identify signs that demonstrate mindful awareness of their boundaries. I also work with clients on maintaining their sense of themselves in time and space because a loss of this sense can represent mindlessness as well as trauma. A hallmark answer that is a clue to therapists that clients may need to do more processing about their exploration is when they answer questions about boundaries and limitations with "I don't know." This answer may not be disqualifying of engaging in exploration, but it's critical to process it with clients to ensure that they're aware of themselves and their boundaries. For clients who have experienced betrayal and trauma, encouraging them to take their time through their exploration journey is also critical.

As you have already probably realized, boundaries can be complicated with all of the various aspects of these relationships. An acronym that can help keep clients grounded is RACK (Risk Aware Consensual Kink). This encourages people to become aware of the risks of engaging in a gathering or activity. It also encourages people to engage in activities that are consensual. No acronym can consider all of the dynamics of these situations, but this is a good start for our clients.

Therapist-Client Relationship and Comfort

Affirming therapy involves increased client comfort in the therapeutic relationship, so they can share different aspects of their life with you. Obviously, this doesn't happen overnight. For clients in this group, it may take even more time. Be patient with this. Remember, it's likely that there is a history of criticism and judgment in this person's life, so this is understandable.

Truthfully, a lot of therapists are uncomfortable talking about sex…period. I've seen several clients who have come to my office because they got the sense that their previous therapist would've preferred to avoid the subject, rather than process issues surrounding sex and sexual desire. For these clients, it might take more time for them to trust your comfort level in discussing their lives in therapy.

Be Transparent

One of the most common mistakes that can cut into trust is when a therapist makes assumptions and pretends. Even with a lot of experience, you're going to have clients who use acronyms and abbreviations, and who identify with lifestyles and arousal that might be unfamiliar to you. Clients don't expect you to know everything, so don't pretend to know what you don't. Just ask! You'll find that most clients will appreciate your efforts to gain knowledge and to understand. On the other hand, if you pretend to know more than you do know, and your client figures this out, it's likely going to be viewed as a form of betrayal.

Helping Clients Who Think They Have an Addiction, but Don't

You're likely to come across clients who think that they have an addiction merely because they have fantasies, desires, or arousal that is taboo in their relationship and/or society. Others might just have a lot of shame around this. Normalization and education, along with shame resilience, are critical when working with these clients.

Timing is everything. If you educate too much, too soon, you risk being condescending to your clients. You can also invalidate them if they're in a struggle, which can push them out of therapy.

Family and relationship therapy are often necessary to help our clients rebuild bridges in their relationships. Sometimes, clients may shame their partners about their desires or arousal. It's important to remember that partners aren't usually trying to be blatantly shameful. Instead, they're responding to their emotions and experiences. Relationship therapy can be an invaluable tool. I've witnessed many relationships get better from couples' therapy.

Remember to give clients time, safety, and space. Again, other aspects of our clients' lives can be impacted by this part of who they are. Just like working with clients who are wanting SOCE, you need to allow clients to share their perspectives. This includes negative feelings such as shame and disgust. When clients have a place to be open, they can work through their feelings, while also trusting your normalization. In time, they're likely to find arenas where they can be authentic, while finding support and possibly even community.

No Assumptions and Letting Clients Draw the Lines

It's crucial that we avoid drawing the lines and boundaries for our clients. When we interject with boundaries that we identify as ideal, we're assisting them in ways that are best for us. Just remember, we're not the ones in the relationship!

As therapists, our role when working with any relationship is to help these clients decide on their own boundary systems. We can provide them with strategies on how to adequately communicate these systems. Some couples may negotiate new expressions of desire. Therapists have to allow this to take place.

Education is beneficial for all members of any relationship. This can include information about boundaries, shame, vulnerability, and authenticity. It may include education about non-traditional relationships as well. I've provided information on these topics by using gentle curiosity. I don't make assumptions, instead I inquire and ask. By approaching this in a gentle way, I am able to break down assumptions and help people see that increased communication isn't a threat to safety and trust.

When we utilize education and gentle questioning, we model open communication. We can reinforce that our clients should also avoid making assumptions. This can also help them identify "deal-breakers" and discuss them. Finally, this approach helps our clients learn background information about boundaries, which is important when negotiating in relationships.

I recommend that clients create a written contract or agreement when they're negotiating new elements of kink, BDSM, and "fetishes." This is particularly important when there are extreme power dynamics in the relationship or in sexual encounters. These agreements can help maintain consensual and safe play in the relationship and prevent abusive situations. It can also help in anticipating what is and isn't okay to our clients.

If you're going to work with clients who are needing your help at this stage of their journey, please do research on how to assist in developing contracts of these boundaries. There are great educational resources where you can get information. There are also many wonderful, experienced sex therapists with whom you can consult.

5

Considerations for Non-Monogamy

Clients who are in open, swinging and polyamorous relationships are vulnerable to shaming that is similar to the other groups mentioned in this book. They can face serious judgment inside and outside of the therapy office. Therapists regularly label non-monogamy as morally wrong. There are also misunderstandings about non-monogamy that lead to judgment and assumptions from our society as a whole.

Unfortunately, the people who come into therapy are often dealing with the fallout that comes from non-consensual non-monogamy. Therapists are at risk of overidentifying these situations as addictions. Even worse, some are labeled as addicts for merely considering non-monogamy in their lives. To be sex positive, therapists need to encourage discussions about monogamy and non-monogamy, rather than avoid them. Transparency and discussion should always be encouraged and treated as bravery in therapy.

When working with these clients, there are several things that therapists have to consider. Again, helping our clients with shame resilience is important. Several of the clients who come into our offices have already stepped outside of monogamous boundaries. These situations are often filled with secrecy, dishonesty, cheating, and affairs. Only a portion of these people are actually dealing with a sexual addiction; yet, the crises that these clients are facing can push them to overidentify with the sex addiction label.

> **There Isn't Just One Person for Everyone**
>
> Traditionally, our culture treats relationships as though we all have one person out there who we are meant to be with. This person is to meet all of our relationship and sexuality needs. Renowned sexuality expert and author Esther Perel has done a lot to break down these myths in her groundbreaking book, *Mating in Captivity*. In this book, Perel discusses how we have evolved from a species that needed to "mate" for survival. Over time, we have transformed into a culture that wants love and commitment in relationships, along with passion and romance.
>
> When I talk with my clients, it seems as though few actually believe that there is only one person for each of us. Yet our society continues to treat love and romance as if people should live in this way. I'm not advocating for any particular relationship structure. I believe we have to take an open position to help our clients. Especially for our poly, open, and swinging relationship clients.
>
> Monogamy is an option. Our culture often views it as the only option, but it's not. Our clients need to understand why they're in the relationship structures they've chosen and why this is what they want. This is true when they enter into non-monogamy, but they also need to know this about themselves when they're in monogamous relationships.

> It can be scary for our clients when we ask them these questions. They may be faced with answering a question that makes them feel uncomfortable. It can also be very empowering. For those who want monogamous relationships, this information can encourage their involvement. Rather than feeling powerless and stuck, these questions can orient people to their goals.
>
> For those who don't view monogamy as the relationship structure that fits their needs, discussing the "one person for everyone" myth can still help. These discussions can promote validation and shame resilience. Dialogue can also help them process their desires with their partners. This helps clients accept limitations, while viewing relationship improvements as a team effort, rather than one person's responsibility.

Even those who are living with compulsivity may desire an open relationship, swinging, or a more polyamorous relationship structure later in their recovery. Unfortunately, there are therapists who treat open discussions about relationship boundaries as if they're a sign of addictive behavior. Clients are often told that it's impossible to balance an addiction and live in an open, polyamorous, or swinging relationship. I can say with confidence that I've watched several clients with addictions grow to a place where they can enjoy trusting non-monogamous relationships.

Helping clients who have a history of betrayal in their relationships navigate into non-monogamous relationships can be quite complicated. But it's important to note that it's entirely possible to make this work when non-monogamy is mutually agreed upon. Clients who are considering these relationship structures often look to the therapist for answers. Sometimes clients even want their therapists to tell them what they should do and what they want. Therapists can guide them with options, but the answers have to come from the clients. I'll be discussing different dynamics and ways of offering support through your clients' journeys throughout this chapter.

Boundaries, Relationships, and Communication

For those who decide to enter into a non-monogamous relationship structure, boundaries and communication are at the top of the list of important relationship considerations. When people come into therapy, they usually want to get right into decision-making and negotiations. They often want to know how to identify what their boundary agreements should look like. However, many clients struggle with defining their boundary systems. This increases the risk of miscommunication and future issues. This is especially true in non-monogamy.

For relationship-building to take place, our clients have to know themselves. I'm not saying that couples' therapy shouldn't occur when clients are confused. Sometimes there is confusion about needs and boundaries in couples' therapy. Some clients have little understanding of their boundaries. This lack of awareness is especially common in our clients who are more likely to have experienced betrayal, affairs, and infidelity as their introductions to non-monogamy.

There are three situations where I believe clients can benefit from individual therapy before engaging in relationship therapy:

1. When we ask clients about their boundaries and they repeatedly answer with, "I don't know."
2. When clients repeatedly engage in a behavior pattern and they report that they don't want to engage in it.
3. When clients ignore personal boundaries in order to satisfy their partner(s).

If you're working with a client and any of these things are true, I've found relationship and couples therapy to be of limited value. It can help people build some relationship skills. At the same time, there is an internal process in these clients that needs to happen. They likely need to increase their self-awareness and build their boundary systems. Individual therapy offers a space for these things to build.

Couples therapy certainly has its place in non-monogamy. Several of the couples who come into therapy for non-monogamy have already explored this. For many of these couples, their problems are based in a lack of established boundaries. In these situations, clients often already had a history of experimenting with non-monogamy to see if their boundaries would emerge from exploring this. It's important for therapists to be patient and understanding in these situations. Relationships often struggle and trust usually decreases when clients are this unclear. Individual and couples' therapy can help clients rebuild trust, while also deepening their personal understanding of their boundaries.

Communication Skills in Non-monogamy

Solid communication skills are crucial to make non-monogamy work. When people come to therapy, they often believe they have the basics of good communication down, when they don't. For example, I can easily recall several clients who told me in their first sessions, "We don't need to work on communication. We just need to figure out what we're going to do with our relationship." More often than not, poor communication is a root cause of their problems.

It can be quite tricky for therapists to help clients manage communication issues when they're resistant of dealing with these problems. When clients come into therapy and don't want to work on communication, we're presented with a challenging dynamic. Ultimately, client goals should be left up to the client. Still, we also have a responsibility to educate our clients about potential problems. When clients are extremely resistant to communication work in therapy, they may need real-time examples of how their communication is failing. Therapy can provide evidence that they need help with situations where their communication is struggling.

I've found The Gottman Institute's communication strategies useful when helping clients learn about the importance of communication. Utilizing Gottman approaches has allowed me to cite some research and offer basic communication strategies. These simple techniques tend to increase client confidence in communication work in therapy. They're often much less resistant when they're able to see the benefits of different ways of approaching conversations.

Sometimes clients will refuse to work on communication no matter what education you offer them. In many of those situations, I've seen several problems occur, which includes the following:

- Shaming each other.
- Being overly critical.

- Hanging out in contempt.
- Feeling entitled to lie or cheat.
- Ignoring the other's needs.
- Using passive aggressiveness to get their way.
- Reactively responding to the other person.
- Living with a lack of boundaries.

This is just a small list of what can go wrong when communication skills are missing in non-monogamous relationships! As you can see, this list is a foundation for toxicity. Therefore, it's necessary to help the relationship build a solid foundation. It's important to educate clients about these foundational issues, so that they're more likely to see the value in this work. When clients accept the importance of building solid communication strategies, we can help them navigate through the issues in the list above. When they don't accept this, we can at least give them information to consider when they face complicated situations down the road.

Ongoing Problems in Non-Monogamy

Some clients will work on their communication, but continue to have ongoing relationship problems in a non-monogamous structure. In these situations, I've found that there are a few primary reasons why they continue to struggle. Look for these problems in your clients' relationships, so you can address them as needed.

1. The people in the relationship continue to struggle with boundaries.

They don't identify their deal-breakers. They might mix up deal breaking boundaries and treat them as if they're negotiable. This will lead to resentment and increase the probability of negative interactions.

2. A struggle with sociocultural issues.

Many clients struggle to identify what they truly want. Those who were raised in rigid and highly judgmental homes also regularly grapple with these cultural issues. Therefore, they can struggle to separate their own needs and desires from cultural messages that they have been taught.

3. Trauma reactivity.

The idea of non-monogamy can be a source of trauma for several of our clients. This will be discussed further in this chapter. I've found that negotiation can only occur when trauma and any history of gaslighting has been processed in therapy.

Boundaries

When working with consensual non-monogamy, boundaries are the cornerstone of success and thus need to be a primary focus of therapy. Whether or not the couple is dealing with sexual compulsivity, a solid understanding of boundaries is always important. We have to be cautious about how we present this topic to our clients. While boundaries can seem easy to understand on the surface, putting them into action is quite complicated.

"I want to explore relationships with other people, but it's not okay if you do."

Some of our non-monogamous clients are in situations that are unfair. The boundaries are set up in a way that one person wants the opportunity to explore romantic and/or sexual relationships with people outside of a primary relationship, while the other one is expected to remain monogamous. In my experiences, these types of imbalanced expectations are disproportionately placed upon women in heterosexual relationships.

Some of these imbalanced situations are set into motion by cheating and affairs. There was no initial discussion about changing the relationship structure and boundaries. Therefore, the relationship focuses heavily on the person who cheated, their desires, and their relationship needs, rather than everyone in the relationship. I've worked with several relationships where cheating occurred, and the husband wants to continue the relationship, but admits he doesn't want his wife to explore other relationships.

Some clients make choices about wanting to remain monogamous while in a relationship with a non-monogamous partner, while some are treated as if they shouldn't have a choice about their relationship structures. I've found these situations especially challenging for me to remain grounded. I want options to be fair in these relationships. I also know I'm not the only one experiencing this because I've heard other therapists talk about their desire for the same.

At the same time, we have to help our clients identify the structure that works best for them. Some of our clients are fine with imbalanced relationship structures. Others focus heavily on their partners' boundaries when they struggle to name their own limitations. In situations where cheating has occurred, this struggle can be related to shock from the trauma of the betrayal. Other times it's purely related to a double standard. Regardless, we have to help them identify a consensual agreement that works for them and matches their boundaries.

I recommend utilizing the *gentle curiosity* approach that I discussed in the LGBTQ chapter. This approach will allow clients to explore their boundaries with you, while not feeling judged for wanting monogamy or polyamory in their situation. Similar to other groups that I've discussed in this book, people may not consider polyamory until they're unexpectedly faced with it. This approach can help clients identify how balanced they want their own boundaries to be.

Game Playing

Boundaries can be quite scary when people are in long-term relationships. They can determine the difference between staying in a relationship and leaving. Although our clients often want to stay in their relationship, some come to identify that their relationship is unworkable during therapy. Thus, the stakes can be high in the conversations they have inside and outside of our offices. Some clients avoid these risks by staying far away from these tough conversations.

One of the common negative outcomes of this avoidance is "game playing." When clients identify their boundaries, it can make them feel incredibly vulnerable. It's natural to search for ways of avoiding this vulnerability. Game playing is one strategy to avoid this vulnerability. This strategy can play out in many different ways. For example, people might attempt to decode their partners' wants and needs rather than assess their own. This way, they don't have to deal with the discomfort of naming and holding to their boundaries.

I liken this strategy to moving a chess piece forward to see how the other person will respond in the game. This is purely a reactive position. There are no cooperative plans, nor are there open, grounded conversations in these situations. Instead, people are just seeing how their partners respond to various interactions.

There is often a lack of awareness of personal boundaries that come with these games, which can often lead to further relationship toxicity. Just because a person is unaware of their boundaries doesn't mean that they don't exist. Some of our boundaries are based in thought and we're consciously aware of them. Others are beneath the surface and are more complicated to identify. Our boundaries are built on our histories and our backgrounds. Regardless of whether they are solidified or not, they're still within us. Unfortunately, this can mean that their boundaries can be repeatedly violated without us recognizing or addressing them. When unrecognized boundaries go unaddressed, resentment is the outcome.

The other problem with games is that they often involve secrets. Snooping is common in these situations. When people snoop, they're looking for information that can prove that they should distrust. When people play games, they're not trusting their partners, nor are they trusting the vulnerability that goes with open communication. Therefore, they don't tell partners that they're snooping behind the scenes. These types of games can enhance betrayal and resentment on both sides. They can also set up unfair expectations about honesty.

Manipulation as a Sign of Other Struggles

I have to disclose a human services pet peeve of mine because I think it's critically important in our work with our clients. I believe this pet peeve is an important consideration that can help us understand relationship games. In all of my years of work in various human service settings, I've heard professionals label clients as "manipulative." It's not necessarily the label that I take issue with, but it's what follows the label that is most problematic.

When we label clients as manipulative, it often leads to client mistreatment. It's as if this label gives us a right to ignore the origins of the manipulation. I've seen clients get dismissed, ignored, openly criticized, and judged after therapists give them this label.

This doesn't mean that the label isn't accurate, but it's important to be mindful of how labels change our interactions. Manipulation rarely is the end of the story. There are almost always vulnerability struggles and unmet needs that accompany it.

Obviously, some people don't care at all about who they hurt. This isn't the case for most of our clients. When they're manipulative, there is usually a deeper story that we need to understand and help them understand.

Deal-Breakers and Negotiables

When considering boundaries, the first line I recommend for people to draw is the one between *deal-breakers* and *negotiables*. Deal-breakers are lines that mean the relationship will have to end if they continue to be crossed. Negotiables are things that are disliked, but they can be negotiated and worked on.

In dealing with intense issues such as betrayal, cheating, and sexual compulsivity, drawing these lines is one of the most important things that our clients need to do. It can also be one of the most challenging things for them to do. When people are betrayed, they tend to react intensely to the betrayal. People can respond to fear, emotional pain, and insecurities in these situations.

Over the years, I've found that clients are often reluctant to name their boundaries. One reason for this is that there is a fear that establishing boundaries will lead to the end of the relationship. This is why I work to slow the process down. I remind clients that identifying a deal-breaker doesn't mean that the relationship must now end. Instead, it means that the relationship needs to focus on understanding and communication.

Boundaries are broad and complicated. Our clients often need time to deepen and understand them. They may also need time to find the courage to tolerate the discomfort that comes with establishing them. Drawing the first lines can be uncomfortable and scary. At first, things will often get more contentious in our clients' relationships when boundaries are established. Then, when clients have a solid sense of their boundaries, they can then identify the options they have. They can discuss boundaries openly, as well as the feelings behind them. Discussions such as these will allow them to further process what is and isn't negotiable.

The Importance of Grounding and Foundational Support

Grounding is one of the most important skills to teach any non-monogamous couple who has a history of infidelity. It can be tough to have these conversations when there has been a history that includes cheating. Listening skills are a crucial component to any relationship. But consider, for a partner who has been cheated on, listening to a story about non-monogamy can be one of the most difficult things to do.

Grounding and containment can also be difficult for someone who has cheated. That person may respond with defensiveness that is mixed with irritation. I've worked with a lot of people who have cheated who respond to discussions by simply shutting down. Without grounding, clients won't be able to talk about their desires, needs, and wants. Most therapists are familiar with grounding, while others aren't as comfortable with it. For a simple-to-use guide to grounding, please visit the website *vantagepointdallascounseling.com*.

Intense emotions are common when cheating has taken place. When there is a sex addiction, the traumas that can come with an addiction can lead to communication problems such as shutting down, attacking, contempt, and defensiveness. It can take a lot of time for people to work through these communication issues, but the time and effort are worth it. It's critical that they learn how to do it. Clients have to learn how to navigate through this vulnerable arena to see what they need to negotiate.

I believe the intensity in discussions about non-monogamy comes from fear, defensiveness about vulnerability, and even trauma. All of these elements can make it difficult to stay in the present. In these situations, these clients are often responding to past threats when discussing the possibility of an open relationship. Those who have cheated may deny their desires out of a fear of what could happen next, but this denial doesn't erase the desires. Instead, it just pushes them back into secrecy and silence, which increases the risk for relationship problems and even addictions.

It's crucial to handle these discussions with betrayed partners with care. Discussing the non-monogamy arena too quickly is one of the biggest mistakes a therapist can make in these situations. When working with betrayed partners, I proceed with extreme caution before questions about non-monogamy. If you ask about this in the wrong manner or if you ask about it too soon, you risk coming across as insensitive. You also risk further traumatizing an already traumatized client. I really work to build a solid rapport and a foundation of trust before I openly discuss non-monogamy with these clients.

Couples need a solid foundation to have these discussions as well. When there has been a history of betrayal, there is a lot of "patchwork" to the foundation of trust that needs to happen before non-monogamy can take place. When cheating has previously occurred, trust foundations will be fractured. Before negotiating anything, the relationship has to regain trust. I'm not saying that trust has to be at 100% to open up meaningful conversations, but if the foundation is only rubble, the conversations are likely to overwhelm the couple and lead to more issues. Therefore, helping the couple patch up their lack of trust before introducing open dialogue about non-monogamy is critical.

Infidelity and Sexual Compulsivity in Non-Monogamy

Some clients come into therapy because they think they have an addiction. Others are pushed by their partners to come in and see us. Some are dealing with genuinely disruptive, compulsive behavior. Others are responding to misunderstandings about non-monogamy. We also have several clients who come into therapy after the discovery of cheating and affairs.

It's important to educate and normalize desires outside of primary relationships. This can scare many monogamous couples, but they aren't dealing with reality when they believe only one person should ever be desired for a lifetime. It's just not realistic. In fact, I believe that denying that reality can increase the likelihood of future problems, including affairs.

Again, when there has been an affair or cheating in your clients' relationships, you have to balance the reality of desires with the pain of a hurt partner. Partners have to regain their footing in their reality. A loss of confidence in intuition becomes part of the gaslighting experience. Re-establishing confidence in intuition and personal experiences doesn't happen overnight.

One way for therapists to approach this balancing act is to determine whether your clients need logic or empathy from you. There is some research that suggests humans have difficulties experiencing both at the same time. In other words, it's difficult to utilize logical thinking when we're experiencing intense emotions. The opposite can be true as well. When we're thinking with extreme logic, it's difficult to practice emotional empathy. Sometimes you need to practice logic with your clients, while other times you need to practice empathy.

A lot of partners need empathy in their relationships, but in their therapy as well. Sadly, many of them get logic when they're in deep emotional turmoil. There is a time and place for the use of education, however we shouldn't be offering education before a partner has had an opportunity to process some of their emotions and grief. It's important to remember that grief doesn't always occur with rational thinking and decision-making.

Therapists can make the mistake of labeling non-monogamy as hypersexuality. This can happen for a variety of reasons. People often assume that those who desire non-monogamy are only focused on sexual relationships. It's true that some people want sexual experiences with different people. Others simply want to experience a different kind of relationship, romance, or love with another person.

Non-Monogamy Doesn't Equal Cheating

People often believe that those in non-monogamous relationships lose their rights to boundaries. I've even heard colleagues insinuate that cheating can't exist in non-monogamy because a couple in therapy enjoyed swinging or had an open relationship. For those who have been hurt and are in non-monogamous relationships, these perspectives can be very harmful.

There isn't anything unethical about consensual non-monogamy. Consensual, open relationships are all about communication and boundaries. These relationship agreements are based in understanding. Of course, it's possible that new challenges may arise in these relationships. Sometimes boundaries are violated in non-monogamous relationships. When this happens, it can cause as much damage as it would in a monogamous relationship.

I believe that assumptions about cheating and boundaries in non-monogamy come from a lack of education. One common misunderstanding is that these relationships are all selfish and hypersexual. In this situation, therapists must learn to identify their biases. Doing so can make all the difference between listening to your clients and hurting them.

Drawing the Lines of Addiction in Non-Monogamy

Again, to identify the lines of compulsivity, we have to help our clients find authenticity and self-acceptance. Although cultural acceptance of open relationships is higher than ever before, we still live in a monogamous-dominated culture. Therefore, many of our clients assume they will always want monogamy. The very thought of non-monogamy can feel like a threat and can lead people to label themselves as addicts.

Deceit and ongoing engagement in unwanted behavior are the prominent signs of an addiction. Those same signs are what you'll look for in cheating and affairs. Therapists have to help their client(s) separate compulsivity from typical cheating and affairs. As you can see, this can be quite a challenge. It can be difficult for those who want non-monogamous relationships to identify and take responsibility for their desire because it's still regarded as culturally taboo in many ways.

Lying

Shame can cause people to lie. In fact, some research shows that lying is a common phenomenon among adults. Lying is generally associated with a discrepancy between how we want people to see us versus reality. Lying in addiction is usually related to a much bigger issue. The disparity in these clients tends to be much more compartmentalized than typical lying.

Lying in addiction can be a powerful and even dissociative force. Sometimes this lying even indicates a significant personality discrepancy. As you can imagine, such a discrepancy can cause significant damage to a relationship. In these situations, partners may feel like they don't even know their partners anymore.

Betrayal, relationship damage, and compartmentalization make lying a critical part of therapy. In situations like these, we have another balance to manage. We have to offer support for the painful experiences of someone who has been betrayed. At the same time, we have to understand the dynamics that lead to the lying.

Women, Non-Monogamy, and Lying

Women in non-monogamous relationship structures can face their own powerful cultural struggles with shame. Our culture comes from a history that has viewed women as possessions rather than individual beings who have their own set of desires and needs. These remnants are still quite powerful in our culture. Today, women aren't only seen as possessions. Instead, they're also seen as people who need to play roles. These expectations can play out in all areas of women's lives, but especially in relationships. Some women want to play these roles, but just as often they want to explore other elements of themselves and their expression. This can lead to severe social consequences. Even outside of non-monogamy, women are often slut-shamed for expressing themselves.

Slut-shaming is the criticism of another person for stepping outside of roles that are assigned by our society and culture. This is primarily a criticism that is reserved for women. Women who want multiple relationships, multiple loves, or who are open about sex are living outside of traditional roles, which may not match up with traditional views of women.

To make things even more challenging, a major source of shame for many women is not being what others expect them to be. There can be serious social consequences for women who don't play these roles. They can face serious judgment. They can lose family support. Some even can lose their children due to cultural misconceptions about non-monogamy.

For women who come from Christian backgrounds, coming out as non-monogamous can come with even more shame. The consequences can be very real for these women as well. Even those who seem to be accepted by their peers can feel very isolated. Women who are non-monogamous and who are from these backgrounds can face suspicion and judgment from friends and family who are supposed to be supportive.

Over the years, I've seen sex-therapists slut-shame women just as much as any other group of therapists. When women express needs or boundaries, slut-shaming is used as a way of cutting right into their power and voices. I've seen weaponry used against women who are wanting non-monogamy, as well as those who don't. Sadly, this behavior goes unaddressed and even buried by professionals and especially professional organizations.

As you can imagine, this increases the risk of lying, cheating and affairs in women. Again, people are responsible for their own behavior, but we also have to be understanding of the cultural contexts that influence behavior. These cultural expectations can influence women to lie and deny themselves of their needs. It also can promote cheating by keeping women in rigid sociocultural structures.

In sessions, therapists can be change agents to this dynamic by holding space for women and encouraging them to identify their own needs. We can also help women by working on shame-resilience. In addition, I believe therapists need to take a bigger role on this issue. I know that my own speaking out about slut-shaming has been buried, ignored, deleted, etc. I will keep speaking out on this cultural dynamic. I hope you'll consider being another voice in this choir.

Primary Relationship Avoidance

Some engage in compulsive detachment in serious relationships. Vulnerability is the pathway to connection, and almost all people need connection in their lives. People who are dealing with addictions struggle with connection and vulnerability as well.

This struggle often creates an incongruence. There is an imbalance of unmet needs, along with a fear of tolerating the vulnerability that is needed to meet these needs. There are often trauma sources that lead to these struggles. Therefore, trauma resolution and vulnerability tolerance are often important focuses in therapy for these clients.

Enhancing Monogamous Satisfaction by Identifying Limitations

Relationship and sexual satisfaction aren't always on the same continuum. Many people are satisfied with their commitment, friendship, and general connection with their partner, while they may also be completely unsatisfied sexually.

For those who want to be in monogamous relationships, they have to contend with relationship limitations. The first step is accepting these challenges and taking responsibility for their part in them. When feelings of sexual boredom, neglect, and frustration occur, personal recognition of the issues is critical. People have to be able to identify their beliefs and opinions around their own lack of satisfaction.

> I encourage people to avoid shame, blame, and comparison in these discussions. When people are feeling sexually frustrated, they're more likely to compare their relationship to the relationships of others. The problem is that this comparison may not even be based in reality.
>
> People can also get passive-aggressive when they're feeling frustrated about sex. This can destroy intimacy and trust. In these situations, there isn't anything to negotiate because relationship concerns haven't even been discussed.
>
> Some people romanticize a past sexual partner who seemed to intuitively know what to do. It can feel like sex is meaningless without this level of intuition. The sad truth is that this level of easy intuitive connection may never exist in a monogamous relationship. It doesn't mean that monogamous sex lives have to be unhappy either. Instead, it merely means that there is more negotiation that will need to take place.
>
> Couples have to talk to each other! So many couples feel uncomfortable talking about sex. It can feel shameful for them to own their desires. Clients can feel like they might hurt their partner if they share their desires as well. This keeps so many people out of this arena. Without talking, there isn't much they can negotiate.

A repeated sense of entitlement is also common in addictive behavior. Rather than tolerating the vulnerability that would come with openness, addicts are more at risk of compartmentalizing the need for authenticity. They can also experience hopelessness in the relationship. Even after a lot of therapeutic work is done, there is usually a long-term tendency to avoid such vulnerability. Thus, vulnerability resilience can help people navigate through conversations about non-monogamy.

Mixing Up Sex, Love, and Boundaries

Some non-monogamous clients confuse sex for love. Obviously, this doesn't only happen with non-monogamous clients. I'm writing about this dynamic in this chapter because I believe that when people struggle to understand their own definitions of love and boundary, they can face some serious challenges in non-monogamy.

When people mix up love, sex, and boundaries, they may engage in things they don't want to engage in. When this happens, relationships are more likely to face chaos because one person ends up being angry at the other person. Yet the boundaries weren't communicated because they were never well-defined to begin with.

I recommend that clients build their own definitions of love, connection, trust, and boundaries. Depending on the client's background, they might need your help to identify a starting point. I recommend building the foundation from the ground up by starting with the most basic boundaries and moving up from there. This means that clients will have to identify elements that are important to them regarding love, relationships, and connection. They they'll have to define these things and figure out how they need to be prioritized.

Diagram

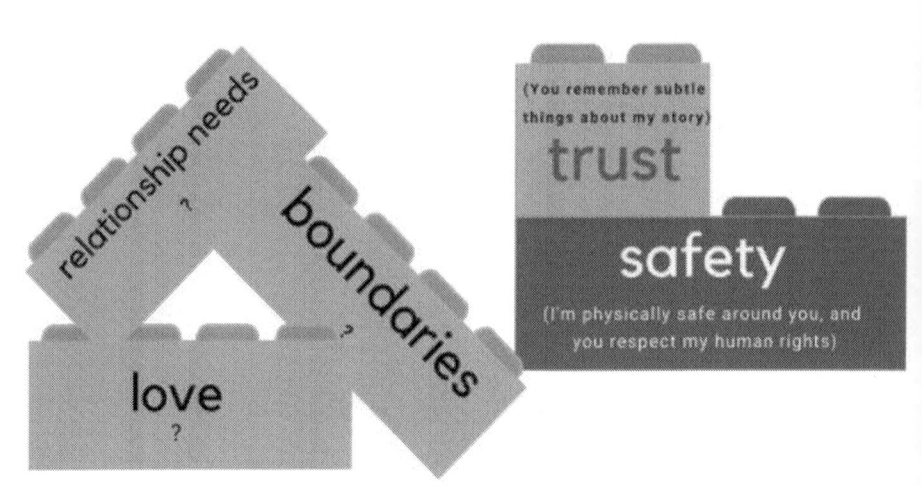

- **relationship needs ?**
- **boundaries ?**
- **love ?**
- **trust** (You remember subtle things about my story)
- **safety** (I'm physically safe around you, and you respect my human rights)

For our clients who had little parental support growing up, the building of this foundation can take a lot of time. For example, it's hard to define trust if your past taught you that you couldn't even expect basic safety in a relationship. We can ask our clients probing questions, or even offer them a list of foundational elements to consider. These things can range from needs, wants, and basic boundaries to any other constructs that our clients need to add in order to achieve greater clarity and personal understanding in their relationships.

Sometimes, clients will have a difficult time coming up with constructs to build their foundation. In these situations, it can be helpful to give them a list to select from. Here is an example of a list they can use to define these things:

Touch	Happiness	Romance
Connection	Joy	Commitment
Eroticism	Intimacy	Fun
Belonging	Passion	Pleasure

This is not a complete list, but something to use to help your clients to identify and define various aspects of their relationships. By taking the time to establish these definitions, they can begin to work on developing boundaries. They'll be better able to recognize when sex and love are combined and when they're separate as well. This process can also help clients avoid simply reacting to their partners' needs. Instead, they can bring their needs to the table and begin the negotiation process.

Shame

As discussed in previous chapters, shame can lead to compulsivity. Those who desire non-monogamy are no exception to this. We have a monogamous-normative culture. People often experience overwhelming shame over sharing their desires with their partners.

When sexual shame is out of control, the person might still explore their curiosity. Rather than people sharing their desires, they're more likely to examine them in secret in this situation. This pattern of secrecy can continue even after discovery. It can also continue after they renegotiate sexual boundaries. It's critical to help clients create a plan to break these cycles when they seek out our help.

As shame builds, people are more likely to numb themselves. Issues with low shame resilience and compartmentalization are going to be more common in those who are at a higher risk of an addiction. Low shame resilience and addiction are a dangerous combination because dishonesty, entitlement, and secrecy are common reactions to shame. Those same reactions can tear our clients' relationships apart.

Leave the Boundary Work to the Clients

At the risk of sounding cynical, I believe it's important to say this. Therapists love to talk about boundaries. I'm including myself in this statement! It makes sense because we realize how important they are in relationships and connection.

Therapists are viewed as boundary "experts" by popular culture. This expert mentality creates a barrier to offering sex-positive therapy. Over the years, I've worked with so many clients who had past therapists who wanted to define their boundaries for them.

There are times where we have to let our clients know that they're breaking boundaries. When they're cheating and lying, or engaging in behavior that is blatantly abusive, we need to educate them about boundaries. It's important to balance this education by offering a non-judgmental perspective that promotes a safe relationship.

Most of our clients don't require such advice. The issues that they're dealing with may revolve around boundaries that are less easily defined. This doesn't mean that you won't see potential

> problems brewing before they occur, but our clients usually have to sort out their boundary systems for themselves.
>
> If we step back and think about it, this is true in our own lives as well. All of the lines that we create come from our past experiences. Our clients are the same. They learn from first-hand experiences, as well as successes and failures. They build their boundaries around these experiences.
>
> When therapists dictate boundaries, it communicates that therapists know best. This superiority can unnecessarily shame one member of the relationship, while advocating for another. Please remain aware of when you *need* to give advice versus when you *want* to give it. If you don't need to give advice, it's better to help the couple open up lines of communication. This allows them to identify their boundaries. After all, they're the ones who have to live with their negotiations.

Sex-Positive Therapy for Non-Monogamy

Because shame and misconceptions are common in non-monogamy, the therapeutic alliance is significant. You may notice trends in themes of attachment, avoidance, and codependency. At the same time, there will be individual nuances that have to be respected. If you fail to appreciate this, you're likely going to lose your client. Even worse, you could shame your clients and cause more harm to their relationship.

You should always pay attention to your assumptions and stereotypes about clients and various relationship structures. Many therapists believe that non-monogamy is always wrong. This can be reflected in the opinions that they share with couples.

Therapists can also push couples into non-monogamy when the couple isn't ready. Non-monogamy isn't the best option when couples are struggling with sexual frustration and poor communication. A lot of people project their relationship frustrations onto their sexuality. Non-monogamy isn't a magic eraser that deletes relationship problems. Therapists should never treat it like it is. Different relationship structures can further expose the problems that already exist in the primary relationship. I tell clients that all of the relationships they're in will have different dynamics and different needs. They have to identify how they're going to manage these dynamics.

It's important for therapists to encourage solid foundations in the relationship. I'm not saying you should never talk about non-monogamy until there is a foundation built. Rather, I'm saying that therapists need to know their place in the discussion. It isn't our job to tell clients to live in any particular relationship structure.

At the same time, it's appropriate to ask clients what they know about non-monogamy and the history of their current relationship structure. I almost always ask my clients how they decided on a monogamous relationship. This is usually followed by a puzzled look because many of them have only ever considered monogamy. Other than those who have been hurt by cheating, very few clients take this question personal. Asking this can orient clients to their options.

Non-Monogamous Bias

Again, there are common assumptions about non-monogamy and monogamy that you want to avoid. Here are some of the common ones that people (and therapists) make regarding various relationship structures:

- Cheating can't happen in non-monogamy.
- Non-monogamy is only for those with a high sex drive.
- Jealousy always occurs in non-monogamy.
- People in monogamous relationships are asking to be cheated on.
- Children will be damaged in non-monogamous relationships.
- Sex addicts can never have a successful non-monogamous relationship.
- Non-monogamy is selfish.
- Monogamy is normal.
- Monogamy is prudish.
- Monogamous couples are more stable than non-monogamous couples.

As is the case in other arenas, we're all likely to hold biases about non-monogamy. The above list doesn't even scratch the surface of where our biases can take us. We live in a culture that normalizes monogamy. Even in the LGBTQ community, where non-monogamy is more normalized, monogamy is still often considered to be "healthier" or "more stable" in many situations.

We must practice ongoing awareness of our potential biases. Once again, this is more than mere tolerance or acceptance of other groups of people. You can accept your non-monogamous clients, while still shaming them! If you have a belief system that monogamy is more "normal," this can be communicated to your client whether you intend to shame them or not.

Relationship Structures and Monogamous Normativity

There are several relationship structures that people can live in. It's important to avoid making assumptions that a monogamous partnership is the goal. Many people who are in non-monogamous relationships have a primary relationship with one person and other relationships as well. Some want equal energy with several partners. Others want some sexual freedom to have sex with other people. There are also swinging relationships, as well as relationships with more than one partner. Beyond these types of relationships, there are countless other structures that people might consider.

It takes a lot of mindfulness to avoid making assumptions. Mindful awareness isn't only something that you must pay attention to at the beginning of therapy either. Needs, desires, and boundaries can shift and change throughout the course of therapy. Therefore, it's important to check in with your clients regularly to see what structure fits best for them.

Sex Addiction and Non-Monogamy

Can sex addicts successfully live in non-monogamous relationships? Yes, they can; however, these relationship structures aren't for all sex addict clients. Some therapists make the mistake of pushing partners into a relationship structure that they don't want. They're driven to believe that the only way to make the relationship successful is to accept non-monogamy. Unfortunately, many of these couples continue to experience the lies and deceit that they had before. Why? Because they didn't address their root issues. They also failed to accept and hold to boundaries in their relationships.

Consensual non-monogamous relationships are different. They involve open feedback and discussions about the needs and desires of people in the relationship. Some partners of sex addicts may shift to feel more open-minded about this type of relationship structure, but many things must be in place prior to this.

First, non-monogamy requires a lot of trust. In relationships with sex addiction, there is often little to no trust. Therefore, these foundations have to be mended to take this step.

There also has to be a solid sense of boundaries. To communicate boundaries, people in the relationship have to identify them. As discussed earlier, many won't know what their boundaries are in the beginning of therapy. This is no place to start non-monogamy.

Before any relationship walks into non-monogamy, the client has to be able to manage the problematic behaviors. If the person goes from addictive behavior to a boundaryless, non-monogamous relationship structure, this will almost always lead to more problems and even more trauma. This doesn't mean that behaviors that are currently out of control can't be enjoyed in a balanced way in the future. People usually just need time and therapeutic work to find this balance.

Finally, clients and partners will have to identify the behaviors that constitute a slip or relapse. The definition of problematic behavior has to be clearly defined. Without these definitions, problems with miscommunication and identification are likely to occur down the road.

As you can see, there can be many challenges for sex addicts and partners who want to establish a non-monogamous relationship style. If these relationships build a solid foundation in their communication, they can succeed at non-monogamy. For this to be a possibility, the couple must have a solid relapse prevention plan, and a period of solid recovery. These definitions will prevent future issues, betrayals, and cheating behaviors.

6

Mindful Sex Addiction Therapy and Beyond

By this point, you have read about various therapeutic considerations for members of vulnerable groups who are dealing with sex addiction. Each group, and more importantly, each individual requires different considerations to successfully help them in a sex positive way. Beyond what I've already discussed, there are other considerations that can help you further fine-tune your approach for each of these clients. In this chapter, I will be discussing various elements that can further help you provide sex-positive therapy to your clients. Hopefully, this information will be helpful whether your clients are dealing with a sex addiction or not.

Sex-positive therapy is a relatively new movement in our field. It's also constantly evolving. New theories and opinions are regularly coming out on how to define sex positivity. In this section, I'm offering my definition of sex positivity because I believe that sex addiction therapy can grow along with this movement.

Sex-Positive Rules

How do you know if you're offering services that are sex positive? I've identified six essential rules that have been critical to the sex positive therapy that I have offered my clients, and I hope that you'll find them useful as well. These rules show how broad the topic of sexuality can be. They include the interpersonal processes of therapists, as well as those of our clients. They contain considerations for personal histories and biases. Finally, they include important demographic factors such as age, gender, sexual orientation, race, and religion.

It's important for me to point out that the information presented on this list of components is very basic. Each one of these topics is so broad, a book could be developed for each of them. For the purposes of this book, I'm focusing on personal considerations for therapists. There is a fluid art to the process of therapy in general. Because sex always involves some level of shame, it can create rigidity that can make the therapeutic process complicated.

Here is a list of rules to help you offer the most sex-positive therapy possible to clients who enter therapy for sex addiction:

Sex-Positive Rule #1: Know and Accept Your Own Biases.

I know I've mentioned this before, but I just can't stress it enough. It's one of the most critical factors in offering sex positive therapy, and guess what? I'm not done talking about it quite yet. Personal understanding of your biases is so important that it earns its own spot on my list of sex-positive rules.

Looking inward to accept your biases is a potentially shameful task. This shame often catches people off guard. The majority of us want to view ourselves as open-minded. This seems to be even more important to many therapists. After all, we're in a field that trains us to accept others for who they are.

I love our field because of its desire to accept others. But sometimes, this desire can overshadow our awareness. It seems like it should be easy to identify our levels of acceptance, but it's often difficult. Remember when I previously discussed the ways that shame can prevent clients from accepting their identities? A similar phenomenon can occur with therapists. Shame can prevent us from being aware of our biases. There is an extreme danger in this lack of recognition. Subtle biases can go unnoticed by therapists and yet clients may still pick up on them.

Ongoing professional training and experience is critical to contend with this. Understanding these biases and how they can impact therapeutic relationships is an ongoing journey. If done correctly, it's never complete. Cultural attitudes and understanding continue to evolve over time. As sexual health professionals, we're expected to know about these changes. Continuing education is one way of remaining aware of cultural changes and following how these changes can impact the therapeutic relationship.

Continuing education can also help us learn about the historical context of our biases and the meaning of their impact on our clients. Gaining a better perspective of our clients' experiences can help us understand them, and it helps us shift our own biases. Otherwise, our clients remain "the other," which still comes with judgment. This type of understanding is critical when empathizing with clients, staying sex positive, and being culturally competent.

Problems with Self-Delusion and Political Correctness

I love that there is political correctness in our society. I believe it helps us identify lines of respect for groups that are different than our own. Unfortunately, in our political climate, the term political correctness has become politicized and even demonized. Once again, the key to paying attention to biases is to remain balanced in an extreme world. Sadly, political correctness has become one more extreme playground to criticize, shame, and judge others.

Here are four of the most common, extreme examples of how I've seen political correctness being misused and misunderstood:

1. You're either perfect in being politically correct or you're labeled an "idiot" or "asshole."
2. If political correctness makes you uncomfortable, you shouldn't have to pay attention to it anymore.
3. Political correctness wouldn't be necessary if people stopped being so sensitive.
4. The dominant culture's struggle is the same as or worse than non-dominant groups.

Political correctness offers some guidance on how to respect and talk about differences. More recently, it has been used to shut down conversations and promote silence. It's been used as weaponry and superiority in various ways. And yes, I've seen these dynamics play out in the sex addiction and sex therapy communities. We can't make progress when we can't talk about issues. We need to create avenues for open discussions, which are sometimes prevented by our shame-based culture.

Shame has also led several people to over-eagerly label themselves as "open-minded." Many refer to themselves as "friendly" to communities of which they aren't a part. "Friendly" and "affirming" aren't the same thing. Friendliness is about the place of business, organization, or person offering the services. Affirmation is about appreciating individual experiences. You can only get to affirmation by accepting the biases that you have.

Even the most "open-minded" people have the potential to shame others without intending to. When professionals fool themselves into believing that they've erased their biases, they're making a huge mistake. They're ignoring flaws, which prevents change from happening. It's tough to own crummy parts of ourselves, but we can't erase these things. We *can* manage them and make them less prevalent when we acknowledge their existence.

It's tempting to try and change in isolation because it's more comfortable. Isolated processing keeps you in your own biases. Biases only change through openness and discussion. Naming and discussing biases can also help you reduce some of your shame when you realize that others are conditioned in the same way. Although it's uncomfortable to walk through these feelings, your abilities in therapy will likely benefit from this.

Sex-Positive Rule #2: Promote Self-Determination.

Most of us have profound knowledge in our specialized fields, but pop psychology has encouraged us to overemphasize our role as life experts. Clients often see therapists play these roles in the media and then believe this is the role they should play in therapy. These expectations have further pressured therapists to act like life experts at times when they don't need to at all. Experts are great on television, radio, podcasts and blogs. Expert advice in therapy is overrated. Therapists need to avoid playing this role as much as possible.

When it comes to vulnerable groups, we have to be even more cautious about stepping into the role of life expert. This is because our culture trains us to view non-dominant subgroups as less intelligent and less capable. When therapists take an unnecessary expert role, they can feed into these cultural dynamics. Our expertise can even lead us to talk right over our clients' fears and boundaries. When we do this, we risk telling them how to handle circumstances that we'll never face ourselves.

The desire to step into the role of expert is understandable. There are times when we need to do it when clients are at a serious risk of hurting themselves. We also need to be directive when clients are in situations where certain harm is impending. Although advice is sometimes needed, therapists often give advice when it's not warranted at all. The timing of advising clients involves complex counseling skills that go way beyond the scope of this book. In dealing with sex addiction, there are times when we have to give advice to help them stabilize crisis situations. Still, we have to provide a safe space for clients to grow and fail as well.

Sex positivity is also about authenticity. We have to help clients identify what gender, life, relationships, and sexuality mean to them. This will reflect a broad spectrum of expressions, orientation, and behavior. Clients need a space where they can process their ideas, fantasies, and perceptions, rather than have them dictated by professionals.

Sex positivity also values all gender expressions and sexual orientations. Gender and sexual orientation occur on a spectrum.

Therapists have to hold space for clients, so they can identify what life, authenticity, and expression look like to them. These things can vary greatly from client to client.

Clients who are trying to understand their LGBTQ authenticity may struggle with religion, coming out, openness in social circles, and problems in their families. We can feel passionate about helping these clients accept themselves. It's important to remember that self-acceptance has to happen on their timeframe, not the therapist's timeframe. Also, self-acceptance often looks different than how we assume it should look in our clients' lives.

There are countless ways in which therapists can interfere with self-determination. There isn't enough room in this section to list them all, but there is one more example that I can't leave unaddressed. Therapists love to define "healthy sexuality." Our field has taken it upon itself to label what is and isn't healthy. There is one primary rule that I use to separate healthy from unhealthy. This is that sexual and relationship agreements must be consensual.

It's important to note that when we're working with people who have a history of trauma, therapists have to be aware that consensuality can be more nuanced. For example, trauma can lead people to allow others to harm them. It can also make it difficult for people to identify what they want and what is acceptable to them. I call this a *dissociated consensuality*. The person may technically engage in a consensual experience, but trauma leads to boundary issues from a lack of personal awareness. When working with sex addiction, gaslighting can be a primary source of trauma. Boundaries can become confusing and trauma can even detach people from themselves. We have an important role of helping clients determine their own boundaries and find authentic ways of enforcing them.

When working with addictions, we have a responsibility to gain a lot of information and education about trauma. Therapists tend to both over- and under-diagnose trauma in therapy situations, especially when it comes to kink, BDSM, and non-monogamy. If there is a problem with dissociated consensuality, the client has to identify this for themselves to align with a plan that can change this. Asking tough questions can help them process boundaries and limitations. Grounding work is also beneficial to these clients. When they build these skills, many come to make determinations for themselves. The bottom line is that even when we identify that our clients have loose boundaries from trauma, they will be making the decisions about what they want in their own lives.

Sadly, I've seen therapists project their judgments about sexuality onto their clients. Clients with non-traditional desires are often already struggling with shame. Can kink, "fetishes," BDSM, and poly be healthy? Of course. If a client is grounded in the present, and makes open decisions with another consenting adult, then it's entirely possible.

Sex-Positive Rule #3: Step Away from Binaries and Open Up to Spectrums.

I've touched on this in regard to our politics. Our culture is obsessed with categories. In particular, we tend to promote opposites. It's hard to understand the middle ground, especially when discussing sexuality.

In sexuality and gender, there are labels and identities that are outside of binary categories. Over the years, I've seen bisexuality, queerness, pansexuality, and fluidity dumbfound therapists. Sadly, when people struggle to understand these identities, they often arm up with suspicion and judgment. For example, I've heard both sex therapists and sex addiction therapists struggle to understand bisexuality. I heard one sex therapist ask, "Why can't they just pick one or the other?"

I don't offer this example to shame those who would ask this question. Instead, I am using it as an example of someone getting trapped in extreme binaries. It assumes people have to "choose" between only two options. When an element is outside of these binaries, it can be puzzling and confusing for people who haven't yet stepped outside of binary thinking.

This type of thinking doesn't occur only when people think about sexual orientation and gender. It can also occur with other relationship structures and other topics of sexuality as well. Some people explore minor levels of kinky play, while others want more of a lifestyle change. There are also those who identify with one label, but explore elements of other labels. For example, there are a lot of people who identify as monogamous, yet who occasionally "play" with others. We have to let our clients identify the labels (or lack of them) that best suit their authenticity. Therapists have to step away from their "either/or" thinking and labeling. This isn't an easy thing to do. We're culturally wired to think about things in this way. We are even neurobiologically wired to classify people into groups. In a way, when we holistically think about people, we're overriding what comes natural in our thinking.

It requires a robust and mindful commitment to follow this rule. Even when you put in this effort, you'll likely fail at some point. Don't worry, we're going to talk about handling our dreaded failures in a little bit.

There is a gravitational force that pulls us towards binaries. I've seen this force pull therapists into binary assumptions. This includes therapists who have great intentions. Genders are often wrongfully categorized when we use binary thinking. I've seen therapeutic relationships with clients get destroyed by therapists who refuse to use non-binary labels such as queer, pansexual, etc.

When you start to feel that pull towards two opposite constructs, it's important to check in with yourself. Turn to the client to gain more information about what they're feeling and what labels work best for them. Turn to them to see if they want a label at all. Most importantly, turn to them to give you the language that they need for support.

Sex-Positive Rule #4: Know Your Place in Cultural Competency.

Cultural competency awareness is something that most of us therapists are required to participate in throughout our education. Let's face it—this training is minimal at best. In counselor education programs, we usually learn only basic information and generalizations about various cultures. Our educational programs usually categorize various groups with fairly broad brushes. We can go through our entire college careers without any real understanding of the regional and individual differences of various groups.

Recognizing our limitations is a critical aspect of sex-positive therapy. When these limitations go unrecognized, you're more likely to disrespect your clients. Over the years, this rule has become very personal to me. I've seen demographic groups (including those of which I'm a member) get overshadowed by people who are speaking for them. I love having allies; however, our current political climate has encouraged an environment where people are pontificating about other groups of people, even when those people are trying to speak for themselves in the discussion. Sadly, this pontification is often used to dominate and overshadow people who are in these groups. To make progress, we have to encourage the loudest voices to be the ones that reflect the demographics of various groups. In other words, if you're talking over someone who is part of a demographic group of which you don't belong, this isn't advocacy, it is domination and it is covert oppression.

Overt and covert domination can really have a negative impact on our clients. Time and again, I've heard clients share stories of how their race, gender, sexual orientation, ability, and ethnicity is talked about by people who aren't part of these groups. This often contributes to social and cultural stress. At its worse, it hits on the cultural trauma that these people have experienced.

To overcome this, it's important for us to remain mindful of our roles as therapists. If you identify yourself as a supportive ally of a community of which you're not a part, you can be an advocate. However, being an advocate means that you can't speak over people who are part of that group when they're speaking out. Instead, appreciate their experiences and embrace learning from them.

There are different cultural considerations for various groups regarding their viewpoints about sex. To validate these narratives, you don't have to divorce yourself from your politics altogether. Instead, you have to find ways of remaining cautious so as not to push your beliefs on clients during sessions. It may sound like common sense, but it can be tough, especially when a client is struggling. When we see our clients struggling, we want to help. Sometimes, it seems like the most natural thing to do would be to share our "enlightened" point of view with them. There are times when our perspectives can be validating. There are many other times when this information can make things more frustrating or confusing for their journey.

Sex-Positive Rule #5: When You Screw Up, Own It.

As you've read, identifying the lines for a sexual addiction can be quite complicated and vague. Also, we're dealing with delicate issues in our clients' lives. Vagueness and cultural differences create insecurity in all of us, including therapists. Most of us have good intentions and yet we're still human. Mistakes will happen.

Cultural and social changes occur every day. We also have to account for individual differences in perceptions about cultural differences. Therefore, we can say the wrong thing to our clients, without knowing it. I've noticed this most commonly in working with gender care clients. Using the wrong pronoun can be devastating to a client. What's even more devastating is when therapists misgender someone, yet don't own it.

Gender is only one example of what can go wrong. The best thing we can do when we mess up is let the client know that we're aware we made a mistake. Although it can be vulnerable and intimidating, it can be a validating experience for clients as well. Although we don't get countless screw-ups (at some point our clients will view this as a refusal of accepting their identified labels), many times, clients will be generous. Taking responsibility shows that you value them and their identity.

There are times when we make mistakes and we don't know we did it. If your client shares a frustration with you, try to view this as bravery. It can be tough to hear it, but it's not easy for them to share their frustrations either. When you listen to your clients and appreciate their experiences, they can increase their trust in you. Even more importantly, they will likely increase confidence in themselves.

Sex Positive Rule #6: Hold Sex-Shaming Accountable.

There are several wonderful residential treatment programs, as well as outpatient programs that offer great, sex positive work. Sadly, there are also several organizations that don't offer the same to these vulnerable populations. Some of these programs still offer SOCE. Some are blatant about their SOCE services, while others disguise it. There are also programs that falsely promise to erase non-traditional sexual desire or non-cisgender expression. This is harmful and has no place in our field. It creates a lot of suspicion toward professionals who offer a safe place to their clients.

We have to hold these people and organizations accountable. I've seen these organizations go without consequences, and in some cases I've even seen them propped up. It's important to point out that this has occurred in communities that are supportive of sex addiction treatment, as well as those that aren't. With my own eyes and ears, I've watched sex therapists and anti-sex addiction proponents shame those with sexually transmitted infections and diseases, LGBTQ people, people of color, and women. I've seen sex addiction therapists secretly offer reparative therapy, promise to erase non-traditional sexual desire, and shame people for their gender expression. To move our field forward, this all has to stop.

Even worse, prominent organizations often ignore reports of therapists who offer these services and behave in this way. Some of this is just bureaucracy. It's also uncomfortable to confront therapists about their treatment of clients; however, when we confront those who are mistreating others, we can become change agents in our field.

I also want to note that there is a distinct difference between being a critic and a change agent. When we're acting as critics, we tend to be reactive, we don't get all the facts and we avoid open discussions. Although critics may seem as though they're acting in the best interest of vulnerable groups, they can actually make social progress more difficult for members of these groups. Critics will often disguise themselves as advocates, but they're actually looking to dominate for personal gain.

Being a true change agent involves openness, dialogue, and a clearness of facts. Stepping out of criticism and into the shoes of a change agent sounds simple, but it's difficult. When we're talking about the groups in this book (and beyond), controversies stem from the historical mistreatment of these groups. This history can make people feel passionately reactive. In some situations, this can prevent open discussions and lead to an attack-defend cycle as well. Don't worry, later in this chapter I'll be discussing how to establish boundaries for yourself when you're having these discussions. Conversely, I also want you to identify when you can stay with the conversation because you can promote some change by doing so. It's hard not to feel reactive when we're responding to a history of mistreatment. It's also hard to avoid becoming defensively reactive when we're talking about cultural pain. We are human after all. I know that I've had my own share of episodes of reactivity. When we have these human moments, it's important to circle back and own our reactivity with colleagues who will respect this and take responsibility for themselves.

Everyone in the therapy community holds the responsibility of working towards sex-positive changes. Whether these changes are broad and sweeping, or small and indirectly individual, they're all significant. Take some time and determine how you can be a positive change agent in your therapy communities. It's not only your clients who will benefit, but you'll likely grow from this experience as well.

Other Advanced Considerations

I hope these sex positive rules helped you identify times where you're succeeding, but also things that you need to change. I am now going to discuss other considerations that can further help you in working with sex addiction. These considerations will further focus on mindful awareness of ego, biases, boundaries, and vulnerability.

Know Your Biases

Have you heard this enough in this book yet? Well, biases show up again here. I can't say enough how important it is to identify your own biases. There isn't a "pass/fail" grade for this. Please don't view this as a type of competition or comparison. Instead, practice viewing this as an area of personal growth, which will also help you on your quest towards being a sex-positive therapist.

In order to check in with yourself about variables in sexuality, sexual orientation, and gender, I've compiled a list of questions to help you assess your own biases. This list should never take the place of ongoing consultation and introspection. My hope is that this can be a starting point for you to ask yourself some tough questions to identify where you need to work on your biases.

Take a look at each question and write down your perspectives on each of them. There isn't going to be a list of "right" or "wrong" answers to follow the questions below. Instead, I encourage you to talk with your colleagues about your solutions. Make yourself vulnerable and open up dialogue!

Bias Question List

1. What causes a person to get an STD, including HIV?
2. Why are people gay or lesbian?
3. How do you feel about people who are bisexual?
4. What do you think about religion and sexuality?
5. How should you refer to clients' race and ethnicity? How do you know this?
6. When is physical pain with sex unhealthy?
7. When is pornography unhealthy?
8. How does religion impact your views on sexuality?
9. What is the difference between gender variance and sexual orientation?
10. What is pornography?

11. What causes a "fetish" to develop?
12. In working with any of the groups discussed in this book, when should trauma be a core piece of therapy?
13. What is the most difficult part for you in working with each of these groups?
14. What do you fear most about working with clients in these vulnerable groups?
15. What more do you need to learn to help clients from these groups?
16. What group(s) in the LGBTQ community do you want to work with the least, and why?
17. When should you suggest more open relationship styles or a monogamous relationship structure to your clients?
18. What beliefs would you have about a polyamorous woman of faith? Do you believe this can even happen?

I deliberately left these questions open-ended, because navigating through our own bias is a lifelong journey. Your answers today are likely going to be different than they will be down the road. We grow and change as time passes. I hope these questions can help you start this process.

After working through this list, what other questions would you ask yourself? One strategy is to think about questions you would ask other therapists if you were helping them identify their biases. Then ask yourself those same questions. Sometimes, it's easier to step outside of ourselves to get to the questions that are useful for our growth. Write these questions down and do the tough work of identifying the answers

How Do You Manage Biases?

As you can see, there are all types of biases that you can (and will) experience. I recommend that you have a plan of action on how to manage these biases in your practice and your life. Again, step away from the idea that "good" therapists have no biases, while "bad" therapists do have them. That dichotomy is nonsense. Instead, identify your biases and work on them. We're all imperfect, and when we practice managing our biases, it will inevitably reflect in our therapeutic work as well.

Here is a basic plan that you can follow to help you manage biases:

1. **Recognize them.**

    It isn't always easy to identify and own our biases. They can bring us a great deal of shame. But you can't do anything about something that you don't even recognize. That is why I created a bias question list, so you can begin to watch out for them.

2. **Be ready for the unexpected.**

    No matter how much you prepare yourself to help people who are different than you, someone's story will eventually catch you off guard. That is where your colleagues come in. Check in with them and be open if something about a client's story bothers you. With these consultations, you can better identify what bothers you so that you can intervene accordingly.

3. **Own your biases.**

    This sounds obvious, doesn't it? Well, it's not. Many therapists are defensive about exploring this part of themselves. Some can be so defensive that they reach the point of lashing out when questioned about biases. If you're defensive, there may be some truth about insecurities that you're holding. Take some time to look into what makes you defensive. Then, you can identify where you need to take responsibility, apologize, and change.

4. Learn and grow.

This journey never ends if you're on the right path. There is always more to learn and explore. I recommend that you go to trainings, but even more importantly interact with people who are different than you. These experiences can help you inside and outside of the therapy office.

5. Refer as needed.

As helping professionals, successfully helping clients can be a source of pride for therapists, but we can't help everybody. There are those clients who aren't a good match for us, and we need to recognize where to draw this line. Again, some of this can catch you off guard. When you have a good sense of your boundaries, it helps you compile a referral list that you can utilize for those clients who aren't a good fit.

Dealing with the Vulnerability of Your Ego Fences

We all have boundaries and we obviously need them; however, boundaries are different than walls. As you have read in this book, the debates surrounding sex addiction have primarily turned into "right" vs. "wrong" and "good" vs. "bad" types of arguments. These arguments are often about the egos within the field more than they're about truly helping people. They can also be about domination and prestige.

Most professionals are extremely knowledgeable in some arenas and have more to learn in others. There isn't anything wrong with discussing concerns about the validity of theories. It's also important to respect that our field is struggling with problems in research. This is because research has increasingly become a race to prove a point or find an outcome that will create an attention-grabbing headline. The best research encourages future studies and welcomes several differing opinions and points of view.

Similar to theories and research, we can only grow by remaining open to a variety of perspectives. I believe you must be open to a peer-review of your own perspectives in order to be sex positive. Listen to the deeper stories behind your colleagues' opinions. I obviously believe that sex addiction exists. I have several friends and colleagues who don't think the same way. I've grown from discussions with people who disagree with me and I bet you will as well.

Of course, you're going to come across colleagues who are less interested in discussing and who are more interested in shaming, criticizing and dominating. I don't want these people to keep you from learning about perspectives that are different than your own. There will be times when it's just not worth talking further with a colleague about any of these issues. I recommend that you come up with your own rules and boundaries to decipher the difference. To offer an example, here are rules that I use. When these rules are broken, I know that it's no longer worth continuing the discussion.

I will continue to stay with the discussion until the other person:

- Insults my intelligence.
- Critiques my self-awareness.
- Repeatedly changes subjects.
- Colludes with others to shame and dominate.

- Stereotypes a whole group or organization and refuses to look beyond their judgments.

I drew these lines for myself because I realized that conversations wouldn't go anywhere in these circumstances unless I sacrificed what I believed and knew. While belonging can feel good, it doesn't always help our field move forward. These are boundaries that work for me, but they might not work for you. I encourage you to come up with your own list. Doing so can help you enter into difficult conversations, while also practicing self-care.

If you keep looking, you will find colleagues out there who are willing to have these difficult conversations with you. You'll also be shocked to see that many of your assumptions about people who hold different opinions are wrong. This can help you grow, but you're also helping our field grow when you use your energy in this way.

Asking Versus Telling

How do we contend with the pressure of being all-knowing experts? We have to recognize when advice is truly needed. There are times when our clients are in crisis. In these situations, they may need advice to help them smooth out a serious mess. This is especially true of addictions and situations where betrayal has happened. Some of our clients might not know how to protect themselves. We can offer them feedback to help them deal with these situations.

One of my favorite suggestions for clients is to "watch for reactivity." I have worked with so many clients who come into therapy when they're in extreme shame. This emotion is so visceral it can make people go to great lengths to get away from it. I've seen clients attempt a complete personality or relationship makeover early in their therapeutic process to avoid experiencing shame. When clients do this, it's more about doing the right thing for someone else rather than identifying what is authentic to them. The problem is that the client can fade into their own performance.

At the beginning of a crisis, reactivity can help clients and their partners feel more secure; however, I've usually seen this break down over time and lead to various other problems. Reactivity leads to avoidance of vulnerability and true personal responsibility. It skips past needed grief and trauma resolution. When people are reactive, they have a desire for fast resolution, but grief and trauma take time to navigate through.

Clients often come into our offices in extreme relationship crises. Their feelings of reactivity can come with a lot of intense energy when they enter into therapy. They often have a sense of urgency or are even in a panic. When that energy combines with a therapist's desire to help, therapists are at an increased risk of taking on an expert position.

To help myself stay grounded, I regularly reassess how I am approaching the client. I focus on whether I am engaging in an *asking* or *telling* dynamic within the therapeutic relationship. If I approach my client from an *asking* dynamic, I am approaching the situation from a curious perspective. The focus of an *asking* approach is understanding and growth, rather than the therapist requiring a specific outcome.

On the other hand, if I approach a client from a *telling* dynamic, I am telling them what I believe they need to know. In this situation, therapists come from a place of power, expertise, and even superiority. Therapists *tell* because they believe they need to take control in order for the client to make progress.

I believe that remaining mindful about *asking* and *telling* can help you stay grounded in your therapy sessions. To further illustrate the difference, here is how I conceptualize both:

Telling is giving advice, without engaging in much ongoing, open processing with the client. There isn't much to process because the therapist has chosen to sit in the expert seat and has asserted that they know best. Taking the role of expert may be necessary in extreme crises and dangerous situations to find a place of safety. It can also be useful when clients get stuck and struggle to make progress. If used outside of these situations, it's much more likely to be about the therapist's discomfort of working with struggling clients.

Asking is different. When we approach discussions with our clients from an asking mentality, we're curious. We don't necessarily know the "right" answers. We encourage them to decide for themselves. Sure, we have our educational backgrounds to rely upon, but with this approach we avoid acting as all-knowing experts. Instead, we are practicing the importance of empathy, experience, and validation.

There are various situations where both approaches can be useful. For example, a client may need to process through their situation with your supportive curiosity (asking). At the same time, they may be stuck in a processing loop that continues to lead to an ongoing struggle. You may offer some education (telling) to help them over the hump and then you can step back into the role of curiosity and validation.

Cases of sexual addiction, problems with sexual arousal, and sexual dysfunction require that our clients learn about their sexuality. In these cases, clients often require education. Though, if we focus too heavily on telling clients what to do, the problems are rarely changed by our knowledge alone. Trust me, I've tried. Being the expert would be so much easier, but it just doesn't work to stay in that position. Sometimes being an expert might work for a little while, but the changes usually only last for a short period of time.

Telling and Labeling of Partners

Please bear with me because this is going to be a critical, uncomfortable discussion point. But I think it's necessary as well. *Telling* is used too often when working with partners of sex addicts. In fact, some of the most detrimental outcomes in therapy that I've seen involved partners of sex addicts. They're another vulnerable group involving sex addiction cases because many of them are dealing with traumatic betrayal, fear, and shame.

Therapists can become very activated by the pain that these clients are experiencing. This can lead them to sit firmly in an expert position. I've witnessed therapists push these clients into assigning labels onto their relationships, partners, and even themselves. In fact, therapists sometimes insist on assigning labels for people whom they haven't even met!

When we misuse labels, we're ignoring the power we have with partners. These situations can quickly blow up in the face of the partner and even destroy the whole family. I've witnessed several examples of therapists misusing their *telling* position with partners of sex addicts. Here are some of those examples:
- "Your husband is an addict and will always act out and relapse."

- "Your partner is abusive and that means…"
- "Your partner is a narcissist…"
- "Your partner is borderline…"
- "Your partner is selfish…"
- "Your husband is gay…"
- "You're codependent…"
- "You're rigid and controlling…"

Of course, there are situations that are entirely unsafe and crises where therapists must intervene. Some clients need safety planning. In those situations, clients may need expert information and guidance. But where is the line?

There are far too many situations where therapists push their own boundaries onto their clients. It's important to allow clients to establish their own labels and boundaries. When we don't let clients establish these things for themselves, we risk damaging the relationship even further. I believe they also can make partners' journeys even more painful and complicated.

I'm not trying to sound critical. I get it. Therapists are passionate about helping their clients. It's understandable to want to help them. I even understand the desire of wanting to protect them. At the same time, they're making their life choices, and we have to respect that. This sometimes means that our clients choose partners we don't like or relationship structures that we wouldn't choose for ourselves.

It's so important to remain mindful. In an instant, we can say something that we can't take back. That information can spiral, especially for someone who is dealing with trauma. When it comes to working with partners, please ask yourself if an *asking* or *telling*

> approach is needed. If you're unclear, please talk with a therapist who has a lot of experience working with partners.

Know Your Professional Limitations

This might go without saying, but I truly believe that sexual compulsivity and sex therapy require specialized training. For sexual compulsivity, there are various ways of gaining proper training. I highly recommend that you get training or supervision in sexual compulsivity, regardless of your opinions about sex addiction. Without this experience, you're much more likely to push your beliefs about sex addiction onto your clients and cause more harm.

I've seen a lot of bad stuff happen when therapists don't have a good understanding of sexual compulsivity. Unfortunately, there are therapists out there who work with sexual compulsivity when they aren't equipped to do so. They shame and label their clients as bad people. Others co-conspire to gaslight hurt partners by telling them that nothing is wrong or by minimizing the impact of cheating.

Some therapists tell a client that there is no such thing as sex addiction. If you feel it's inappropriate to use addiction terminology when dealing with sexuality, be cautious about how you proceed with your clients. Telling a person that addiction doesn't exist comes with risks. Some clients are dealing with compulsivity and don't want to face this. When a professional has told them that their problem doesn't exist, it can validate that denial. This cuts right into the reality of those around that client and makes that client's journey even more difficult.

Unfortunately, I've seen therapists offer sex therapy for sexual dysfunction with little to no training as well. These services are often uninformed, which can lead to serious problems such as increased shame, frustration, and confusion. Sexual dysfunction can occur from a variety of issues including physiological, mental, emotional, and spiritual dilemmas. If you don't have education in these issues, you can negatively reinforce the source of the problem. I highly recommend you find a sex therapist or educator who offers training to help you gain essential knowledge on these issues. Otherwise, it's best to refer to someone who has this experience.

Acknowledging limitations can be tricky. Sex addiction and sexual dysfunction often go hand-in-hand. For example, I've worked with a lot of clients who were dealing with issues of premature ejaculation and erectile dysfunction, as well as porn addiction. I've also worked with several partners of addicts who contend with low sexual desire. Trauma, fear of vulnerability, and issues with connection can all increase the risk of sexual problems.

When sex addiction and sexual dysfunction concerns overlap, I recommend a couple of things. First, I recommend a temporary separation of concerns. Truthfully, several of the sexual and relational issues that our clients are dealing with are likely interrelated. Without a little separation, though, they can become a jumbled, confusing, and overwhelming mess. This can lead to confusion of boundaries and needs. It can push our clients into a place of reactivity.

When our clients can separate their issues, they can better prioritize their focus. They can process and intervene in different arenas. Processing doesn't have to be rushed. Instead, our clients can ground themselves, focus on different aspects of their lives and then bring all of these things back together. Mindfully approaching various issues makes negotiating much more manageable.

Finally, I also recommend consultation. Find a therapist who has experience working with these overlapping issues to help where your experience is lacking. This can include finding a sex addiction therapist or sex therapist to consult with. Fortunately, there are many sex addiction and sex therapists out there who are excellent resources.

Accepting Client Struggles as Growth

Accepting our clients for who they are and where they're at on their journey is one of the most challenging things for therapists to do. This difficulty can come from good intentions. We want our clients to do well. Therapists have to remain mindful to provide a space where clients can build their own identities and discover their own goals.

There is a word that therapists love to use that can counter self-determination. It's also a word that I believe we have to walk away from. The word is "resistant." Although clients can be resistant, there are personalized reasons why this is happening. In my experience, this word is often used as another way to dismiss clients. I've even heard this word used as an insinuation that some clients don't "deserve" help. For the most part, when clients show up in our offices, they're working on themselves on some level.

I try to view defensiveness and resistance as opportunities for growth and understanding for our clients. I also recognize that these issues are often difficult for us to help clients navigate through. When someone takes a defensive stance, it's natural to respond from a critical position. I find that consultation and centering help me stay grounded when I am helping a client work through challenging topics and processes.

We all go through processes of change in our lives. We move through ebbs and flows during these times. Sometimes there will be progress, and other times there will be steps backwards. Sometimes it might be difficult for our clients to identify what progress even is to them.

When working with any issue, there are times when we might need to push on the edges of the narrative to help the client move. Clients need gentle, yet firm approaches when dealing with compulsive behavior. This is a balance. When therapists aren't gentle enough, shame and avoidance can occur. When therapists aren't firm enough, they can triangulate and collude.

For therapists who are tempted to push too quickly, too soon, I offer the following metaphor. Imagine that you want to buy a pair of shoes. The clerk asks you if you need help and so you give him a stern look, and say "I'm just looking." If the clerk continues to insist that you need to buy a new pair of shoes, and you're not ready to make a purchase, you're likely going to leave the store.

Many of our clients are "just browsing" when they first come to therapy. They often begin their work with us because of outside influences. It's up to our clients to decide what needs to be changed in their own lives. Therapists can offer support, curiosity, and validation, but clients decide when they're ready to make a purchase.

Mindfulness and Centering

As a therapist who is trained in Somatic Experiencing, I know that even a self-aware bunch like us mental health and addiction therapists can struggle with mindfulness. Trust me when I say that I'm not being critical of this because I've traveled my own journey of growth in mindfulness as well. Our lack of mindfulness can even be further impacted by shame. Again, owning our biases can cause a pretty intense level of shame, which can take us out of our own grounded sense of mindful awareness and leave us feeling reactive.

Shame can quickly make us lose ourselves in space and time. It can transform us from empathetic therapists into critics who are defensive and shut down. It can take us away from our present tasks of supporting and helping our clients navigate through complicated life circumstances.

I know that shame isn't the only emotion that has the potential to be triggering to us during sessions. We can experience a wide array of feelings that can interfere with our therapy sessions. Although shame may be the most intense emotion, all emotions and feelings can impact us. What do you do about it? I recommend learning how to center yourself.

What is Centering?

Centering is an approach that can help you prepare yourself (in mind and body) for what may happen next. There are always unknowns when we work with clients. At the same time, some things are more likely to occur in session than others. Some of these situations are challenging. Centering can help us prepare for these situations.

Centering involves taking some time to prepare yourself mentally and physiologically for what's coming next. Taking some time before all sessions can be helpful. It can be especially beneficial when working with clients who have issues with sex and relationships. When you give yourself time to center, surprising therapeutic situations are less likely to negatively impact you. You'll be better able to respond in a way that promotes client growth and empathy. It can also help you prepare for those cases that you identify as challenging. Keep in mind that some of the most challenging cases can include those clients who you want to help the most.

Here is how centering is done. Give yourself a few minutes before the session. This requires planning and holding onto time boundaries for sessions. I do 50-minute sessions and will use those 10 minutes before the next therapeutic hour to center when I need to. In that time, practice self-talk that helps you feel prepared for the upcoming session. Use this self-talk to get yourself ready for the next session. You can use this time to offer yourself helpful reminders or you can also use it to reestablish boundaries.

Here are some of my favorite self-talk strategies to center myself:

- "This client could really shock me today."
- "This may be an intense session, but I know I can handle it."
- "This is my client's journey, not mine."
- "I can help."
- "I have a lot of good experience."
- "I can be there to support this client."

No matter what I choose to say to myself, it's a preparation for the session to come. It also helps me identify emotions that could become an issue. When I recognize the potential for problematic emotions before the session, it prepares me so that I can contain and manage them as needed when they arise. I can also consult with peers about my clinical struggles because I have identified them.

The last part of centering is a scanning of your body. I regularly scan my body for any visible signs of tension, anxiety, or tightness. If these things exist, I will literally shake, flex or clench to help the tension move and shift in my body. This doesn't get rid of the emotion, but helps me prepare for the work ahead. I always ask myself, "Are you prepared to work with this client?" I've never answered this negatively, but I find that it helps me remain grounded.

Centering Practice

It never ceases to amaze me how much practice centering can take. In fact, the practice is an ongoing process. You will change as time goes on. Your perspectives and even boundaries can change too. Over time, you may become bothered by new things. In other words, if you're doing it right, the practice of centering never ends.

Following is a list of questions that I ask myself on a regular basis to practice centering. I hope you'll come up with your own list of questions too.

Centering Questions:
- How are you feeling about the work?
- How are you feeling about your client?
- How prepared are you for this client?
- What emotions do you notice now?
- Are you able to hold space for your client?

I also need to mention that body awareness is another critical part of this practice. Sometimes our mental perspective doesn't match the story of our bodies. There is an incongruence. Your mind might say that you're comfortable, but your body may reveal that you're tight and tense. This is why I recommend that you also take some time to check in with your body. If you feel tense and tight while you think that you're comfortable, you might want to work on body-based mindfulness and awareness. I recommend that you explore this with another professional who is skilled in body-based therapies.

In order to notice centering in your body, you'll need time to get more practice under your belt. When you get better at it, you'll identify trends in your sensations that signal particular emotions. You'll also become better at finding balance with internal resources. Finally, you'll notice a series of sensations that signal contentment, or even sensations that help you get to a deactivated place before a session.

Here is a simple exercise to get you started with practicing centered body-awareness:

1. Bring up an image of a client case.
2. Let the image gently dissipate.
3. Notice what sensations appear in your body.

Then ask yourself the following:

4. What makes you feel the most confident?
5. What changes in your body?
6. What makes you feel the calmest about this case?
7. What changes in your body?

> The goal of the last step is to find what makes you feel the most deactivated. When you focus on a series of sensations associated with deactivation, you'll be able to use them to identify a centered place from within your body more quickly. This practice can increase your overall sense of congruence.

Boundaries and Sex Positivity

If you notice that you're continuously struggling with a client, it may mean that you need to spend more time processing your boundaries. First, you need to give yourself time to care for yourself during the day. I know that it's easier said than done. I've struggled with it too. It's important to schedule time for self-care, centering, and reflection. Find peers who will hold you accountable and ask you about this.

Boundaries are also important when working with your clients in session. Sometimes therapists want to help when their clients aren't ready to make changes. Our responses reflect our level of comfort and connection with our clients. Can you recognize the separation between you and your client in session? Does it feel like you're two separate beings? When we're working with complex issues and trauma, it can be difficult to turn to these questions in session.

We all hold boundary-based energy that surrounds and protects us. The most obvious example of this boundary is our skin. However, our boundaries extend well beyond that. We're surrounded by a protective unseen layer of protective energy as well. We need to practice awareness of this energy and identify how it impacts those around us. For example, I want to protect myself, but I also want to leave room for clients to share their stories. If the energy outside of myself is too big (and sometimes it is), it can encompass the whole office. This doesn't encourage my clients to share in an open way. I also want to avoid absorbing too much of my clients' stories and energy. There is a balance and it's essential to remain aware of how expansive your boundaries are in each session.

When therapists fail to identify their sense of boundary, they can send off unconscious signals to their clients. Those who have a history of trauma are sensitive to the energy of others. Clients who come into therapy for issues with sex and sexuality regularly have a history of trauma. This is true of those who are dealing with sexual compulsivity as well. Trauma is also very common in those who are part of the vulnerable groups discussed throughout this book.

Mindful Approaches for Client Sensitivity

Addicts are typically very sensitive people. This can be quite difficult for therapists to believe. Every client with addictions has a high probability to come into therapy with situations of betrayal, lies, and distrust. When we see these clients, we typically have someone who is sitting in front of us who has hurt many other people. Sometimes it's difficult to see their sensitivity through the betrayal and boundary crossing that has occurred. As you get to know your client, you'll see it emerge more over time. When this sensitivity is mixed with poor coping skills, the foundation is built for cycles of addiction.

This isn't to say that people aren't responsible for their behavior. Managing this responsibility is a critical aspect of the recovery process. This can only occur with an increased tolerance to negative emotions. I believe that increased awareness, acceptance, and appreciation of personal sensitivity are critical in changing these cycles as well.

Shame Resilience

Poor emotional resilience increases the risk of client attrition. Those who seek out therapy are likely to use defense mechanisms to cope with conflict, discomfort, and self-evaluation. They might block out, shut down, avoid, or become belligerent against the therapist. They might claim that they don't care about what others think. These mechanisms can be a barrier for therapists, but they can also be a gateway for building client rapport. When a therapist is able to connect with these experiences, client retention tends to increase. Over time, the therapeutic process can help the client build ego-strength and shame resilience. The client will also better tolerate looking into the mirror that is held up during the therapy process.

To help build this gateway, sex-positive therapy must involve shame resilience work. Again, shame resiliency is important in all therapy, but it's especially important in sex addiction cases. It's even more important in cases with members of vulnerable populations. Therefore, when we notice our clients' defense mechanisms, it's likely that they're connected to shame in some way.

To help build resilience, clients and therapists must understand shame. First, it's important to recognize when shame is present, even when nothing wrong has been done. We tend to think of it as an outcome of negative behavior or a stepping outside of our own values system. Shame also prevents us from doing and saying things that might express levels of authenticity. It's that internal voice that reminds us that we may not be worthy of certain types of attention, that we might not be accepted, or that who we are and how we feel is wrong. These feelings can prevent us from taking chances.

The source of our shame comes from our need for connection. Because we often learn tough lessons about shame, we build up defenses that help us disconnect from the pain of the feeling. Almost all of the addicts with whom I work have extreme sensitivity to what others think and feel about them. There are all kinds of defenses that can be used to deal with this. Therapists can help clients understand these mechanisms and the role that shame has in their lives.

Reactivity and Emotional Awareness

Intense emotional experiences can lead clients to become reactive. When people cross a threshold of pain, they work to get out of it. There are strong, visceral feelings associated with difficult situations. However, most of us have adequate coping skills to manage these situations. Many of our clients lack these skills. Therapists must monitor for client reactivity and use it as a tool for therapeutic growth.

Reactivity is seen in several different forms. A client might jump into therapy with an intense energy. They might seek advice to "sort everything out," only to become bored with therapy after a couple of weeks, and then develop a strong desire to quit a week later. They might want to "just get out" of their marriage because they can't handle a partner who is hurt or angry. They also might make promises that they can't keep, hoping to make their partners feel better. Therapists have to blend in techniques that help clients remain interested in therapy. We also have to help our clients learn how to regulate themselves. Self-regulation will go a long way when they're faced with the harsh realities of how difficult it is to deal with complicated situations and negative emotions.

Acceptance of Connection Failures

Connection isn't easy to establish, reestablish or maintain. It reflects a survival instinct that is wired deep within us. Addicts regularly struggle with this need. You will see this struggle come out in the form of shame and reactivity in therapy. It can also be seen in their emotional struggles before therapy. Throughout the therapeutic process, clients can learn that connection includes a felt sense that can be extremely positive. At the same time, finding authentic connection involves surviving several episodes of failure, working through tough emotional times and managing conflict with empathy and reciprocity.

Orientation to the Positive

Orientation towards positive experiences can help clients work on their tolerance of the intensity that comes with negative experiences and feelings. Therapy can focus on unpacking triggers and personal narratives, but sometimes the focus can become too negative. Addicts are commonly out of touch with negative emotions, but they can also be out of touch with positive emotions. They can struggle to identify what positive emotions exist and how they feel in their everyday lives. This positive focus can help clients create pathways that increase identification with other experiences.

Gentle Confrontation

Gentle confrontation can help clients tolerate the process of looking into their experiences and lives. I've found that confronting our clients in the right way can promote them to look deeper into themselves. Some clients generally avoid this type of introspection, but they might be more willing to explore these things with a gentle push. In fact, clients often welcome a little confrontation. It keeps therapy engaging and thought-provoking. It also encourages clients to think further about what was discussed in session, which is important for ongoing introspection.

In a therapeutic confrontation, the balance is very delicate. When pushed too far, the client can be shamed and disengage from the therapeutic process. To facilitate a balance, therapists need to provide a space where clients can remain skeptical about their therapists' perspectives. When they're encouraged to be open, it can model healthy disagreements. This is an experiential opportunity that many clients have rarely had in their lives.

Self-Compassion

Self-compassion can help clients manage shame and emotional reactivity. Although many of our client cases can include painful life decisions and mistakes, they can still find a space for personal understanding.

There are a number of clients who will insist that self-compassion can be dangerous. It's important to educate these clients that there is a difference between self-compassion and self-enabling. Self-compassion is a look at the underlying causes of the behavior. Enabling is about making excuses for the behavior. Clients don't have to give up self-compassion in order to succeed. In fact, I don't believe that they can succeed without practicing it.

When to Embrace Labels and When to Leave Them Behind

The psychotherapy field is filled with labels. Whether it's the diagnoses or the schemas that we use to quickly understand our clients, labels matter. As you're probably aware at this point in this book, I focus a lot of attention on giving them up, but they do have some value in our work. When we use labels, we can quickly identify trends in behavior, which can help us anticipate and prepare for our clients' needs. As you read in the section on centering, preparation is extremely important.

Labels can also give therapists a common language. When we're processing a case with our colleagues, we need a way of conveying the dynamics of the case to our peers. Without using any labels, the case can become difficult to share. Therefore, labels can help us ask the right questions of our colleagues. In fact, they can even help us ask the right questions in session.

Labels are everywhere in the therapy world. There are diagnostic labels in our field, but ethnic, racial, gender, religious, and sexual orientation labels can be relevant to our clients too. Outside of diagnostic labels, there are several other ways that therapists use labels and schemas. They can help us quickly synthesize and interpret information. Unfortunately, they can also stigmatize clients and lead to shame. In working with sex addiction, we have a responsibility to know when and how labels can stigmatize and when they're useful and necessary.

In my many years of experience, I can say that not all clients are shamed by labels. Some identify with labels. For example, the addiction label can help some people find support in their communities. Race, ethnicity and sexual orientation labels can help people make sense of their own stories. There are countless other ways that labels can help our clients. When therapists disrespect these labels, they can interfere with their clients' growth and processing.

> **Embrace the Vague**
>
> Therapists often over-rely on labels because they can create an illusion of control. Labels can give therapists a sense of certainty. They make it seem like there is one "correct way" of helping the people who sit with us in therapy. This sense of control isn't real. There is no linear pathway to helping any client. People are complicated. Moods, perceptions, and life circumstances are likely to change throughout the therapeutic process.
>
> I encourage therapists to embrace some vagueness. There will be many situations where you won't know what label best fits your client. There will also be situations where your client won't know what labels they identify with as well. Rather than focusing your attention on labels, I recommend that you allow this to collaboratively unfold with your client. Your clinical opinion matters, but your clients' opinions matter even more because it's their life stories. Your reassurance can help clients use their self-determination and build a more solid sense of themselves.
>
> It would be wonderful to have a specific roadmap that would help direct us on how to help each client. However, each of our clients will have a different story to share. I believe that diagnosing has its place in therapy. I also believe that it's limited in its usefulness. Our clients are more complicated than the diagnoses, constructs and social categories that we use to understand them. There is no map that makes helping people easy. When we appreciate our clients' individuality, we will face vagueness in every case.

> I know that vagueness can leave therapists feeling very vulnerable and even insecure. We can be a perfectionistic bunch of professionals. We want our clients to do well, but there is a caveat. Our egos can also become tied to our clients' success. Sadly, therapists are sometimes the ones who label success and failure for their clients. I believe that the over-emphasis of labels can feed into our egos. When we become trapped by our egos, we lose touch of the subtle processes of therapy. We also risk forgetting about the power of validation, openness, and the therapeutic bond.

This isn't to say that labels never cause problems. As you have read throughout this book, labels can lead to a variety of issues. They can oversimplify our clients' lives. When we use labels to oversimplify people, this promotes dichotomies in treatment such as:

- Right vs. wrong
- Good vs. bad
- Always vs. never

Let me use sex addiction as an example. If I make the statement, "Sex addicts always need church and prayer in their lives," I may not be reflecting certain clients' needs. In this statement, it's the therapist who is determining the needs. In another example, if I make the statement, "You should never use the label of sex addiction because it doesn't exist," I'm at risk of ignoring certain clients' stories.

We can't reduce our clients down to whether they're dealing with an addiction or not, or whether they're dealing with depression or not, etc. In other words, labels are there for therapists (and insurance companies) and their usefulness is limited. Our clients' stories matter. Not just parts of their stories, but the whole thing. Sometimes their stories are messy. Other times they're confusing. Listening to them with an open heart and mind may create cognitive dissonance in our minds. We have to stay alert to this dissonance and deal with it accordingly. This can be frustrating, uncomfortable and exhausting. When you're maintaining a balanced perspective on labels, you'll feel all of these things at some point when working with your clients.

Conclusion

I hope that by this point in this book, you have gained information that can help you with cases of clients who are vulnerable of being mislabeled as sex addicts. I know the water can be muddy and sometimes it can even feel less clear as you continue to gain more knowledge and information. Sexuality and gender are complicated. When you mix in the complexities of culture, shame, and personal values and beliefs, diagnosing a problem always becomes complex and confusing. Sex addiction is just one example of how complicated sex and diagnosis can be.

I began this book by discussing the controversies surrounding sex addiction. I'm sure that many therapists who read this were already aware of these controversies. I covered this because I think it's important to discuss the controversies from different opinions and perspectives. I hope that I represented different perspectives well and that this helped you understand opinions that are different than your own.

Regardless of the controversies surrounding sex addiction, my focus has always been on helping the people who are brave enough to work with me in therapy. Sadly, the debate on sexually compulsive behavior has pushed our field further away from this. It has become more about competing professional opinions, attention, and domination. Our clients are often left confused as a result. In worse-case scenarios, their experiences are debunked in a way that has harmed their relationships and made their journeys more difficult. All therapists hold responsibility for this.

I believe the key to helping vulnerable groups is mindful self-awareness in therapists. When therapists aren't causing direct harm to their clients (i.e., offering SOCE), then discussions and processing should take center stage. At this time the show is dominated by overreaching generalizations about professionals whom are different. This has been especially true of the sex addiction debate. It's unfair to therapists to make such generalizations, but it also negatively impacts our clients. It prevents the advancement of treatment for these groups because it prevents open discussion. Rather than therapists coming together, the division gets bigger by blame, slander, and criticism.

Over the years, the most alarming professional display that I've seen in therapists involves the misuse of marginalization for personal gain. When we're talking about the marginalization of various groups, we're all responsible for the structures that hold oppressing systems in place. If you're pointing a finger without asking how you've contributed to the oppression, you're contributing to oppression, discrimination, and bias by ignoring your part in all of these things. I hope this book stimulates thought about your personal responsibility in these systems.

There are more than two sides to the discussion on sex addiction. Unfortunately, our field has made it seem like there are only two sides of this issue: "believers" and "deniers." The landscape has been painted as if everyone has to choose a side. This is inconsiderate. There are several sides to this debate.

I don't shame the voices who've been loudest on this topic either. I respect their passion about this. Passion is often the only thing that brings awareness to issues. These voices also bring a broader attention to problems that involve sexuality and gender. Increased awareness allows us to reflect while challenging professional theories and ideas.

Debate is healthy when it doesn't resort to shaming and demonizing someone who has a different perspective. It's uncomfortable to hold such a space. I hope this book can serve as a point of ongoing discussion. I also hope that it serves as a grounding force to keep us focused on how important it is to talk with professionals who have differing opinions. I know it's easy for passion to take over in these discussions. When discussions turn to domination, shaming, and criticism, own your part. Circle back, apologize and try again.

I recognize the fact that our field continues to change and shift. It has changed a lot since I became a therapist. This book is in no way complete. Groups such as sex workers also deserve attention when it comes to sex addiction treatment. Race, ethnicity, gender, disability and many other cultural considerations deserve much broader discussion than what I've covered in this book. There are also a lot of elements regarding sex-positive therapy in the families and partners of sex addicts that weren't covered in this book with the depth that they deserve. I look forward to future books and literature that focus on the impact on other groups that weren't discussed in this book.

Lastly, I hope this book serves as a reminder of the importance of listening and respecting individual stories. Our clients' stories will vary greatly, regardless of whether they're dealing with sex addiction or not. That is where the art lies. It's the art that helps people.

References and Resources

Alvavi, S. S., Ferdosi, M., Jannatifard, F., Eslami, M., Alaghemandan, H., & Setare, M. (2012). 2012. *International Journal of Preventative Medicine, 3*(4), 290-294.

American Psychiatric Association. (2000). *Diagnostic and Statistical Manual of Mental Disorders* (Vols. 4th Edition, TR). Arlington, VA: American Psychiatric Publishing.

Association, A. P. (2013). *Diagnostic and Statistical Manual of Mental Disorders* (Vol. 5th Edition). Washington, DC: American Psychiatric Publishing.

Autri, S. (2014). *What you need to know about hypersexuality.* Retrieved from AASECT: https://www.aasect.org/what-you-need-know-about-hypersexuality

Brown, B. (2012). *Daring Greatly: How the Courage to Be Vulnerable Transforms the Way We Live, Love, Parent, and Lead.* New York, NY: Gotham Books.

Carnes, P. (2009). *Recovery Zone.* Carefree, AZ: Gentle Path Press.

Carnes, P. (2015). *Facing the Shadow* (Vol. 3rd Edition). Gentle Path Press.

Conover, P. (2002). *Transgender Good News.* Silver Springs, MD: New Wineskins Press.

Dyer, T. (2016). The Existence, Causes and Solutions of Gender Bias in the Diagnosis of Personality Disorders. *4*(1).

Enlightenment, I. f. (n.d.). Retrieved from https://instituteforsexuality.com

Grant, J. M., Mottet, L. A., Tanis, J., Herman, J. L., Harrison, J., & Keisling, M. (2010). *National Transgender Discrimination Survey Report on Health and Health Care.*

Green, J. (2004). *Becoming a Visible Man.* Nashviller, TN: Vanderbilt University Press.

Griffith, S. (2014, 12-February). *Strong religious beliefs may drive self-perception of being addicted to online pornography.* Retrieved 2015, 2-August from Think: http://blog.case.edu/think/2014/02/12/strong_religious_beliefs_may_drive_selfperception_of_being_addicted_to_online_pornography

Grubbs, J. B., Exline, J. J., Pargament, K. L., Hook, J. N., & Carlisle, R. D. (2015). Transgression as Addiction: Religiosity and Moral Dispproval as Predictors of Perceived Addiction to Pornography. *Archives of Sexual Behavior, 44*(1), 125-136.

Hardy, J. W., & Easton, D. (2017). *The Ethical Slut: A Practical Guide to Polyamory, Open Relationships, and Other Freedoms in Sex and Love* (3rd ed.). Berkeley, CA.

Institute, T. G. (2016). *Gottman-Rapoport Conflict Blueprint.* Retrieved from The Gottman Institute: https://www.gottman.com/wp-content/uploads/2016/09/Money-Conflict-Blueprint.pdf

Katehakis, A. (2016). *Sex Addiction as Affect Dysregulation: A Neurobiologically Informed Holistic Treatment.* New York, NY: W. W. Norton.

Katehakis, A. (2016). *Sex Addiction as Affect Dysregulation: A Neurobiology Informed Holistic Treatment.* New York, NY: W.W. Norton & Company.

Khoury, B., Langer, E. J., & Pagnini, F. (2014). The DSM: Mindful Science or Mindless Power? *Frontiers in Psychology, 5*, 602.

Kort, J. (2018). *LGBTQ Clients in Therapy: Clinical Issues and Treatment.* New York, NY: W.W. Norton & Company.

Medicine, A. S. (2011). *Definition of Addiction.* Retrieved from ASAM: https://www.asam.org/for-the-public/definition-of-addiction

Novella, S. (2013). *DSM-5 and the fight for the Heart of Psychiatry.* Retrieved from Science Based Medicine : https://sciencebasedmedicine.org/dsm-5-and-the-fight-for-the-heart-of-psychiatry/

Ogden, G. (2013). *Expanding the Practice of Sex Therapy: An Integrative Model for Exploring Intimacy.* New York, NY: Routledge.

Perel, E. (2007). *Mating in Captivity: Unlocking Erotic Intelligence.* New York, NY: Harper Paperbacks.

Perel, E. (2017). *5 Assumptions People Always Get WRONG About Long-Term Love.* Retrieved from http://www.yourtango.com/experts/esther-perel/5-mistaken-assumptions-about-long-term-love-expert

Sanchez, F. J. (2016). Masculinity Issues Among Gay, Bisexual, and Transgender Men. In J. Y. Wong, & S. R. Wester (Eds.), *APA Handbook of Men and Masculinities* (pp. 339-356). Washington, D.C.: American Psychological Association.

Sue, S. (2001). Science, ethnicity and bias - Where have we gone wrong? *American Psychologist, 54*(12), 1070-1077.

University, C. (2016). *What does the scholarly research say about whether conversion therapy can alter sexual orientation without causing harm?* Retrieved from Cornell University: https://whatweknow.inequality.cornell.edu/topics/lgbt-equality/what-does-the-scholarly-research-say-about-whether-conversion-therapy-can-alter-sexual-orientation-without-causing-harm/

Voon, V., Mole, T. B., Banca, P., Porter, L., Morris, L., Mitchell, S., . . . Irvine, M. (2014). Neural correlates of sexual cue reactivity in individuals with and without compulsive sexual behaviours. *PLOS*.

Williams, D., Thomas, J. N., Prior, E. E., & Walters, W. (2015). Introducing a multidisciplinary framework of positive sexuality. *Journal of Positive Sexuality*.

Manufactured by Amazon.ca
Bolton, ON